SAFE IN THE ARMS

Gale Wild

New Generation Publishing

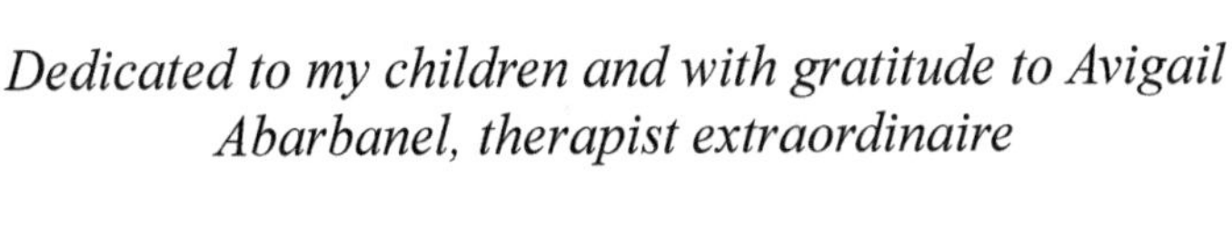

CHAPTER 1

The Stage is Set

Was I the result of deception or delusion? I'll never know. Returning after WW2, not a conquering hero but a traumatised hospital-case and one with a case of syphilis contracted during his military duties, my father informed my mother that he was now unable to father a child. So she took no precautions against parenting a child in such dismal circumstances. Fact is - I appeared and then, fast on my heels, two more, including the longed-for son.

And my father adored me to start with. Of my two older sisters, Margaret, born 1939 and Rose, 1943, he had seen so little that he had not bonded with them at all. But me he took upon his knee from the start, marvelled at my childish utterances and tended to my cuts and bruises. My mother was edged out but was probably only too glad as she seemed unable to connect with anything other than a baby-blob. And she had an ever-expanding brood.

It is not that I judge my mother harshly. I had picked up enough of her dereliction early on. She was the only surviving child of a World War 1 working-class family and aged seven, had heard her own mother lament the fact that it was not she that was 'taken', but her big brother. Daniel had been fifteen when he was kicked in the kidneys playing football and he died a lingering death. Mum's home-life then went downhill, her father took to drinking and her mother had a love-affair.

By the time I was born, Mum lived near her parents but it seemed a miserable connection. By that stage, my seventy-year old granddad was a scary giant of a man, at one time twenty two stone in mass, shut up in the front room, sometimes with his cronies but usually with a bottle. My mother was very bleak in nature understandably and completely unable to show affection. I only remember her laughter a couple of times.

My father, on the other hand, was often full of gaiety but as often in the most vile of moods, with a violent temper. Whether this was due to his war-trauma or not I do not know, though family legend has it that he was always prone to a nasty temper and had really alienated all of his siblings. Born in 1914 to a school-teacher mother, his father had returned home at the end of the war with gas on his lungs and died not long after. Dad was thus reared in a large family by a widow.

It had been an ambitious family and his siblings did well professionally, two of his sisters getting scholarships to Cambridge. Dad failed the Latin part of the entrance exam and did not go to university till after retirement. He landed up working all his life in a routine but secure job as an Executive Officer in the Customs and Excise. This had one compensation for him, in that he chose to work supervising the Excise duty on whisky, which meant his work-location in beautiful countryside and access to free whisky. His lack of academic success had a profound effect on him, however. He pushed us mercilessly to succeed academically where he felt he had failed.

Such two adults, so typical of their era, married in haste before WW2 though in fact Margaret was on the way at the time of the wedding. My mother would have died had this fact been discovered. The wedding anniversary was never marked in any way. I at the time thought that was due to the fact that there was nothing to celebrate about my parents' marriage but I suspect now it was because the date would have given away my mother's guilty secret. She had had to get married. All my teenage years and beyond she ranted on nevertheless with great venom about any unfortunate girl or young woman who also fell into this plight, she vehemently denounced how awful the shame was for their mothers. But the fact is that she herself ran off to get married in Gretna Green against the wishes of her father who disliked my father intensely and denounced him as 'mad.'

Such a marriage did not produce a home fit for children and was rent with violent rows. Of which more later. This took a horrible toll on us and I woke all during my childhood from the age of four on with a terrible dread. Was Dad in a good mood or not, was he singing or was he cursing my mother for having mislaid his cuff-links. ?

The setting of our home was however idyllic. We lived always on the banks of the beautiful River Spey in the north east of Scotland, at first in a series of rented cottages. And then in 1953, with the aid of a cheap mortgage, the family home was built just outside a little village.

My first five years however were spent in a village nearby, where my grandparents lived till the end of their days. So for those first few years I saw them regularly. My early memories of our gardens, the views from them and the feel of it all was of a magical landscape peopled also with the characters of the many tall tales of my older sister, Rose. And, like kids of our generation, we spent most of our play-hours outdoors.

Also like most kids of the era, we were all subjected to the rigid childrearing methods of the time, strict breast-feeding and weaning schedules, shaming toilet-training and always early to bed. So did this routine over-riding of natural rhythms appeal to my mother's rigid nature that she told me in adulthood with almost a hint of pride of how she weaned me. Apparently my father had in vain pleaded with her to give me the breast when, after three days of refusing the bottle, I was screaming from starvation. My mother had a will of iron and I had to clamp myself on the bottle eventually in desperation, thus beginning, I think, the terrible wall of love/hate I felt for my mother.

My hair was resistant to her desire for a curly silken-haired daughter and she dragged a brush fiercely through my wiry locks in spite of my wails, she primped it with painful curlers and clearly wished me to look like a doll. So I grew up stubbornly a tomboy.

Only once did she pause in her routine – she had me standing on the table whilst she wrestled with my tuggy hair but was required to stop by her ingrained reverence for the fifties establishment. Over the radio boomed a sepulchral voice telling listeners that the 'King was Dead.' A minute's silence was proclaimed.

My mother stopped tormenting my hair, looked grim-faced and sighed, not for loss of her monarch but because Mrs Dale's Diary had been taken off the air as a mark of public respect.

Like all young children I was resilient at first and managed to salvage that sense of living in paradise that is, I believe, our birth-right. My world was magical indeed. And Rose was a large part of that. Nothing was its prosaic self, the wood surrounding our garden was enchanted, we had fairy houses under the beech hedge, the leaves of which she taught me to relish. The big rock in the midst of the street was the tomb-stone of a little boy, chillingly, she added, killed by our very own father. Miss Roy, the nosy parker from across the road, she made the unfortunate victim in many a lurid tragedy. Her fairy-story world became legend in my mind. Without any emotional mothering, Rose became the centre of my daily world till the return of my father from work.

The moment I heard the wheels of his car crunch on the gravel I would rush to meet him. I remember waiting outside on a bench overlooking the Spey with the last inch of an ice cream cone I was saving for him. I adored him and he seemed to adore me. As he left for work he would give me a kiss on the cheek, ignoring my mother and older sisters. Their jealousy was so palpable and understandable to me that it was not long before I wiped away his kisses or chose not to rush to him. Then Margaret and Rose had once quizzed me "Do you like Daddy?" "Yes" I chirruped blithely. "You'll find out" Margaret said darkly. And find out I did.

Firstly there was the result of the parental neglect of Rose on her attitude to myself. From my early years, she understandably was highly ambivalent to me, alternating from frenzied cuddling to punches on the nose. Later on, her angry barb on being required to share a Christmas bike with me ("You always spoil things for me") became an accusation that entwined itself around her plight and later her suicide.

Then there was the volatility of my parents and how she reacted to it. One episode still replays in my mind rent with Rose's screams of agony. We had been bouncing on our beds when we should have been settling to sleep. There was a furious yell and pounding of enraged feet up the stair. The door flew open and my father flung a hot water bottle across the room. Of course, he did not intend for it to hit either of us but it did. It hit Rose's back, burst and scalded her badly. She was rushed to hospital with serious scalds. She had to lie in bed for a week on her tummy covered in bandages and often crying in pain.

No outside intervention followed this – and the only significant response I noticed was going with my mother to the village store to buy Rose a treat - a Korky the Kat annual. It was one of those old-style grocery-stores, it was Christmas, all the old wooden fitments gleamed with polish and wonderful aromas filled the air. A glittering Christmas tree complete with candles dominated the counter. I was truly entranced. Later I remember mum changing Rose's dressings, I saw the red blisters but I was never-the-less jealous that she got the Korky annual and a bit guilty, as if I was somehow to blame or should have been scalded instead. I did pay a price in a different currency however.

Next Hallowe'en, I was sitting on my father's knee by the fire – I was all dressed up in a magical little leaf-green and speckled paper skirt and enjoying being cuddled by my father. I was happy. The door opened and a group of strange figures stood there – my sisters and friends all dressed up. Further delight. But as with all my delightful memories, there was always a black seam. Daddy had been showing me my toy violin which was a small replica of his own and even had a proper bow of gut. I loved it and wanted to play like him. But some time later Rose showed me the bow – it was broken – she told me that Daddy had broken it on her back. I never had a violin again. And never did know how my bow got broken, by Rose in a jealous fit, by accident or in the way Rose told me.

Moreover I was rudely evicted from pride of place in my father's affections with the birth of Ewan when I was four. The birth of my youngest sister, Elizabeth, when I was two and a half was not greeted with displays of family joy. But my father got wildly drunk to celebrate the birth of the long-awaited son. I was demoted and was no longer his pride and joy. Indeed I was now subject to the same abuse as my older sisters. I began to feel awful about myself and paradoxically found consolation in the closeness that developed between myself and my new brother.

My world, however, first truly shattered around my ears at the dinner table, at least that was my first memory of the sudden and terrifying outbursts of maniacal rage that would erupt between my parents. I must have been about four and a half as my little brother was ensconced in a high chair at one end of the table. The ritual signal for hostilities, that was later to become so dreadfully familiar to us kids, began. My father found some reason to begin taunting my mother. I cannot remember what it was on this first occasion but his repertoire included the state of the Sunday joint, her complexion, her fat.

Then across my field of vision streaked my mother, wielding a carving-knife directed at my father. That episode is carved indelibly into my psyche. He must have had quick reflexes because he caught her wrist. She threw herself out of the room yelling "I wish you were dead." On another occasion, she upended a mass of crockery and I was hit on the face by a flying fork. My father rushed to me to soothe my screams and hurled at my mother – "Look what you have done to her." What hurt me most here was that my wound was used by my father to get at my mother. From then on I suppressed any visible display of the terror I felt.

Such brawls punctuated our childhood home periodically and, though there was usually a build-up of tension for a few hours with my father's relentless taunting and nagging my mother, the real onslaught could come at any moment – we never knew when.

Our welfare in all this never seemed to cross my parents' minds, even though my little brother was a baby in the path of the carving knife, sitting trustingly in his high-chair. We inevitably began to suffer, all in different ways. The most visible tragedy was of Rose, whose suicide, aged nineteen, I mark in a special separate testament at the end of my story.

Moreover, looking at this issue of parental standards with adult lenses, I can only conclude that my mother's attitude to our safety was ultra laissez-faire to the point of dangerous. She often left us as toddlers in the care of a very under-age sibling. Thus I was left in my high chair with a three-year old Rose whilst my mother left the house to hurriedly walk the ten minutes there and back to the Post Office. Howling in rage and upset, I turned around and threw my head forward angrily. It crashed through a window I had been left close to. I do not remember being hurt, only Rose getting a dreadful row for not looking after me right. Then again a three-year old Elizabeth was left in a room with an open first-floor window out of which her baby brother climbed and fell, luckily with no injury, into a flower bed.

Because our mother was trying to pretend to be middle-class, we were not permitted friendships with the children around us, who were mostly children of distillery or railway workers. Thus entering primary school was an overwhelming experience for me. In a room with two infant classes and around forty children with quite a fierce teacher, I was terrified. The playground was large and I do remember running around yelling with the others but I did not know how to make friends and all the other children seemed to know each other. So I was a natural target for bullies.

Two girls in particular delighted, whilst walking home, to take me to a sand-pit where their fun was to rub sand in my face. Unable to deal with this, I did nothing, rubbed my face and waited till they had gone – I then cried and ran home. In desperation after a few weeks of this, I found another road home. But a big boy, George, followed me. He pointed at the Broomy Isle in the midst of the black swirling waters of the

River Spey. "You better watch out" he said "there is a wolf running wild down on the isle. My Dad is out trying to shoot it. You had better not go down this road." I took to my heels and once again arrived home in tears. My father spotted me and took notice. The next day I remember my hand in his as he marched me up to the school. He informed the teacher that I was being bullied and it had to stop. And surprisingly it did till we moved house a few weeks later and I started at a new school.

Again it was a girl who tormented me. Agnes lived up the same road as myself and as we walked home she would as often as not turn on me and punch me in the face. I still did not know how to deal with this. Eventually one day I turned tail and ran in tears the half mile back to school. A shy girl, I must have been desperate, propelled by terror to knock at a classroom door where our teacher was still at work with an older class. I blurted out my sorry tale "Agnes Campbell hit me." There was no sympathy, only an expression of bother that I had disturbed her class. And Agnes still kept it up. And then there was Beatrice in the school canteen who bullied me at mealtime under the very eyes of the teachers. No interventions to protect me and I just took it.

Was I lacking in backbone or some essential self-protective instinct? I certainly felt ashamed that I did not know what to do. Moreover I thought that the fact that these girls did not like me was only to be expected. Who had not treated me thus so far in my life? But with the benefit of my years I can see myself as so traumatised by my previous family trials that I was too frozen to react in a healthy way. This only set me up for more poundings.

It is testimony to the power of the human psyche that I somehow managed to learn the basics of primary education. What I really liked at school was the infrequent chance to play with threading shining glass beads, the paper Christmas trees we made, the playground running games. The endless chanting of tables and spelling I endured with the rest of my imprisoned peers. But the main lesson of my schooling, like that of my home, was how to live with fear.

CHAPTER 2

The Second Seven

I have heard it said that the years from seven to fourteen cover the age of latency when a child's inner life, sexuality and turmoil become submerged. Perhaps this could account for the fact that my memory of these years lack the vivid immediacy of earlier times, almost seeming bland by comparison.

We had moved up from our first home when I was six in a small Austin car stuffed with five kids, some of our belongings and some frantically clucking bantam hens. And this meant for me a changing of sleeping companions, starting off sharing with my wee brother, Ewan, then in a room with Elizabeth and Margaret. Then I had a few years with Rose until, when I was about fourteen and Rose had left home, I chose to sleep in splendid isolation up in the attic. Where I slept was key to my emotional welfare and, for my first couple of years in the new house, I was much more secure because I had Ewan to cuddle and love at night and he returned this to me. He was a very soft and trusting little boy.

It was a terrific blow to my security when my childhood bedtime cuddles and capers with Ewan were abruptly cut short by my father. Hearing us laughing together and possibly jealous or perhaps annoyed that I kept Ewan awake telling him silly stories, he announced that I was to move to the bedroom with my sisters because I was, he said, getting too old to sleep with my brother. I interpreted this in a dumbly obscure way as if somehow Ewan and I had been guilty of incest, though I did not know what that was or indeed what sex was. I must have been picking up dark undercurrents in my father's troubled mind, currents which were to be made more conscious later on in my life.

Moreover when he went to school it became increasingly hard to relax or have much fun with Ewan except at bed-time. Suddenly but often, he became sullenly aggressive and shut-down. Years later he told me he got bullied because of my father's foul temper with the distillery workers whose sons were in Ewan's class.

And by this time I shared a room with Elizabeth and Margaret, with neither of whom I felt at all close or safe. They were usually cold and irritable to me. Elizabeth in fact somehow managed to play boss in our childhood games, and, even though she was two and a half years younger than me, I was scared of her coldly fierce tongue. Margaret, being much older than all of us and bearing the brunt of my father's hectoring about helping my mother, had very little care for either of us. In fact she was quite nasty to us. I was so nervous of these sisters' bad temper that I started to be unable to go to sleep.

Being overwrought, I used to have to get up and pee a few times in the evening. Margaret once hurled at me – "What is the matter with you? You must have kidney problems." This rang alarm bells in me and was, I think, supposed to – we were all too aware of the importance of kidneys in relation to Uncle Daniel's death. For a few years after that I had an underlying fear that I would die very soon, not an easy fear to talk about and I told nobody.

Superficially by this time I passed as a quiet docile child with no evidence of problems but about the age of eight, I felt very awful inside. At night, I would line all my stuffed toy animals up along my pillow beside me in bed. Then I would gaze with a sad heart at my favourite, a battered bristly black dog with the most endearing expressive eyes of a deep yellow. Suddenly I would smack him viciously then hurl him out of the bed, telling him he was a bad dog. Then I would lie still in bed thinking of him lying freezing and rejected on the floor. When it all became too much for me, I would burst into tears, jump out of bed, retrieve him, smother him in kisses and comfort-cry myself to sleep. This speak volumes as to how much the harsh punitive energy around me a lot of the time left me bereft and desperately needing to be held and comforted. But by this stage I had closed off from showing any neediness in public.

My diaries are noticeably lacking in any reference to anything drastically wrong at home. Occasionally there are references to my getting a row at school and lots of upbeat chat about the usual trials of childhood, moans about piles of homework in secondary-school but the content of my diaries are very pathetically unemotional, filled with details of my daily life, like what comics I got, when we had rhubarb crumble, which TV programmes we watched – we got a TV when I was about thirteen - and also the name of the many films we say in our local flea-pit cinema or in Elgin – the former all for the sum of six old pennies –

equivalent of five p now, with a penny off if you took back a lemonade bottle.

My father, for all his sins, did notice something was very wrong. One day, as I was trying to sidle out of the dining-room, he was speaking to me and he said "Why can't you look me in the eye anymore?" I said nothing as I did not know I was avoiding his gaze and also because I could not admit to myself, or him, the strength of the fear I had for him. I think I mumbled something and continued to sidle out. It now never ceases to astonish me that he should have wondered at my obvious fear. He was quite capable of suddenly lashing out with a wallop around the face or elsewhere.

One occasion I remember was when he had taken us three youngest children on what was a lovely walk across several fields. By my adult reckoning, it must have been a tramp of at least one mile and we were very weary. He sat us on a dyke for a rest and took a photo of the three of us, grinning trustingly at him, a photo I still have which brings such sadness to my heart. For a minute or two later he wanted us on our feet again to walk home. The two younger ones he had carried part way but I had had to walk what is quite a distance for a child who was then about six. I started to girn. A sudden very hard blow across the side of my head and ear left me reeling. My consciousness exploded behind my eyes and for a few stunned seconds the world was a humming white blank. I almost fell off the wall. I can still feel a burning sense of outrage and shame at such a sudden assault. These sorts of blows were frequent and often, when he had a moment earlier been sunnily laughing. That, coupled with his tendency to long maniacal and tyrannical screaming bouts, made him a terrifying person. So it is no wonder that I would cower from him and from then on, sadly, I would stiffen automatically if anyone came near me.

My feelings for him, however, were, until about ten, highly charged with ambivalence. To illustrate, when I was around nine, he gave us three youngest children a small plot of garden each. He used to garden sometimes beside me. One day he said to me, out of the blue "I don't want you to cry for me when I die." I was outraged and asked him "Why not?" He replied "Because I am a bad person." I was very annoyed with him and said defiantly "I will cry for you" – this shows that I was, still, at that age capable of feeling love for him. But the sad fact is that, when he did die, so many years later, I did not shed a tear. I felt only massive relief that our family hell was over. Had he died when I was a child, however, I think I would have cried. I think it was also on this occasion that he added "I am sorry I am so horrible at times. I try not to be but I really cannot help it." The fact is, I knew he could not.

I have thus not ever been able to feel a healthy anger for my father - it was so laden with the sympathy he created in me by such outpourings. And after the age of ten, I was aware only of a creeping dread of him and of trying to shrink away from him at my seat so close to him at the dining-table. I felt no love for him at all – indeed I hated him.

My mother was no source of comfort for us in all this – on the contrary, though she visited her rages on us less often than my father, the release of her pent-up force was terrifying. On one such occasion, she was walloping my little sister, aged about seven, so fiercely and with such a degree of screamed murderous malevolence that Elizabeth passed out and collapsed on the stairs. I tried to pick up her slumped body. This would not be the last time I had to perform such a sorry duty. And indeed my twelve year old brother had to gather me up off the floor after I collapsed in the teeth of a volley of lethal venom from my mother, only a few days after the death of Rose.

Back to my bedding. How glad I thus was to be eventually moved into the same bed as Rose. She was often very sweet to us younger ones. She read us many a story, cuddling us on her knee. As she did so, she would either twiddle on the ends of her hair or she held a small object she would fondle as she read, one of the more obvious outlets for her nervousness. Sometimes she joined in our games, not often as we were much more childish than she.

However perhaps one of my happiest memories of childhood is of walking in a pine forest in the snow with Rose and Ewan. The sky was blue, snowflakes were flying past Rose's face and she was smiling. It was like the lights were all on in my world. I felt breathtakingly happy to see huge snowflakes drifting past her smiling face, etched against a background of blue sky and swaying pines.

However, given her background wretched state, her often violent outbursts at me meant I could never fully trust or be unreservedly close to Rose. In fact by this age I trusted nobody in my small world.

This time of my life was also, however, one of wider exploration. My father would load us into the car and take us down to Lossie beach on the slightest suggestion of sun. We loved swimming and I would go in and out for a dip several times each trip. This was one of the few settings where my mother seemed to relax. She prepared a huge picnic for us and dished out steaming cups of tea from the vacuum flask, in between swimming strongly herself. Dad also liked to take us on long hikes and pretty soon we would set off on our own without him. We once cycled all the five miles to the base of Ben Duig and climbed nearly all the way up it – all under nine years of age. We made a raft out of old oil-barrels roped together and tried to float it in the Lyme burn, not very successfully. We even waded together across the river Spey, which was probably quite dangerous. Once Ewan got injured when I was leading the gang on a climb up a quarry bank. Elizabeth's foot dislodged a stone and it hit Ewan on the head. We led him bleeding home.

I began to get some friends at school. Delightful Sheila, whose father was a gamekeeper and was also the caretaker of a huge old country mansion, once showed me a hidden room in which there were some genuine swords from olden days. Her mother was very kind and I loved visiting her. We used to run down to her house through a bed of forget-me-nots and often walk half a mile to hang out with a couple of woodcutters. They used to sit us on their knees and give us bites of their pieces, doughnuts and cream buns. Nowadays they would be prime child-abuse suspects but they were probably married men working away from home and missing their own wee ones. I was really devastated when Sheila's parents moved away when I was eight.

Then to a cottage just up the road along came two boys, Robbie and Billy, both younger than myself.

They, with Elizabeth, Ewan and myself, became a little gang of five. In spite of being painfully shy and quiet at school, my real mettle came out in this setting and I was their unquestioned gang-leader. Though Robbie was only a few months younger than me, I could wrestle him to the ground and was thus top-dog.

As a gang we roamed far and wide and adopted a posture of belligerency towards the world outside our homes, aided by outfitting ourselves in old WW2 steel helmets and gas-masks. We had catapults and bows and arrows. We hid in our tree-stump hiding-place and yelled insults at the passing gamekeepers whom we hated. They used to snarl at us for walking on the riverbank and allegedly disturbing the fishing of their wealthy paymasters. We did hoaxes like packing up smart looking parcels full of rubbish but written on them was "Evidence for the Great Train Robbery." We would leave the parcels on the road then watch what happened from behind our hedge. It was very breath-taking seeing cars stop and people exclaiming over our parcels. A few of our packages did indeed land up at the police station. And we did get a gentle warning from our local bobby who obviously was soft on practical jokers.

On a more domestic side we built our own houses, presumably in an effort to feel some sense of our power. The father of the boys was a pompous tyrant who used to beat Billy for wetting his bed. It was horrible to listen to. He was a teacher at a local orphanage and sometimes took a couple of the boys up to his home for a visit. I watched him raise red weals on the bare legs of a lad who had run about the garden with his seed-dispenser unwittingly sowing things where they should not have been.

Our alternative play-homes, however, bore a strong resemblance to our real abodes in key ways – Robbie and I lay in a field discussing with relish how we would punish our children. We lighted on a big stone over which our future offspring would have to lean as we meted out their just punishments - we called this the spanking-stone. Somehow I retained my authority over this little gang in spite of being a girl, though I do remember feeling very awkward when my breasts stated to grow - I could no longer run about with just my shorts on as I had been used to.

Then sadly the parents of the boys left to live some way away and this coincided with my moving up to secondary school so it was another gloomy milestone. From then on I became, or attempted to become, one of the girls and never more had boys as friends or roamed so widely and freely on foot, though I covered miles by bike.

The rows between my parents still raged, though their impact on my memory is blunted and not sharp. And in fact my father did make efforts at this time to be a 'good father' He organised us regularly to play cricket, made us a table-tennis table and a dartboard complete with brand new darts. He always arranged huge Guy Fawkes bonfires for us and our neighbours and Mum would bake tatties for the occasion. In this era, the fifth of November was not a big celebration in Speyside so a good few kids came and this was really fun. My father seemed to like the fiery element.

Both parents also seemed to come alive whenever there was a big storm. No doubt being of stormy natures, the dramatic weather-events spoke to their deeper selves. I remember once the snow was so deep that we had to walk down the drive in Dad's footprints or be carried. And of going to school with huge snowdrifts on either side of the road. Moreover one year there was a terrific gale which wrenched trees up by the roots – and even according to my father lifted up an old lady up the Rinnachat road and deposited her on the other side of the road. The night of the big wind liberated my mother briefly from her dogged obedience to her martyred compliance to domestic routines. She was forced to take time just to be with us at night. With no electricity we younger kids crouched with her in her bed by the light of a candle, listening to the wind batter the house outside, the only occasion in my childhood when I remember feeling cosy and safe with an adult. Perhaps I have blocked memories of any others.

Dad also organised family holidays for us – often a week in a caravan on Nairn beach. Again my mother was usually in a good mood then and there were fun times as we just swam all day and ate ice-creams and had lots of chips. One year we ventured as far as Ullapool although the camp-site had a black hole for a toilet and left much to be desired. We often spent time with families with whom my parents were friendly. As my mother was a snob, this involved us being taken to learn to ski with richer family friends, to skate on a local pond or to visit at their homes. These also were good times though I was always dimly aware that my father flirted openly and outrageously with many of the women involved and that he and the men absented themselves for periods at the pub or drank a lot in the evenings. This was before the drink-and–drive laws were changed so Dad often drove us home in a very drunken state.

School was something of a nightmare apart from the games in the playground. Out of my six primary school teachers, four were absolute monsters, terrifying all of us. I remember aged seven innocently passing a scissors to one of my teachers. As I was ignorant of safety rules, she bawled my head off for handing them to her point first. I do not know how I learnt anything as I was not able to concentrate much of the time in the class-room, I was so pre-occupied. In P4 however there was respite and I had a few months with Miss White, who was kind and gentle. I developed a passionate crush on her and day-dreams where she was my doting mother. I was jealous beyond measure when she left to get married.

I had other crushes following on this, firstly for a girl slightly older than myself. My attempts to get her attention were rather counter-productive as I would follow behind her from school and shout silly things. Eventually she had had enough, grabbed my school beret and threw it over a wall into someone's garden. I never did get it back, much to the annoyance of my mother. My beret was supposed to mark me out as a cut-above the other 'common' children.

The next few objects of my fantasies were boys who had some glaring problems like being fostered or having a brother who stuttered. They clearly would need me. Then later in secondary school I fell for older boys who did not spare my class a second glance, or for the more handsome of our male teachers, whom I placed in the role of adoring father. All this gave colour to my life, even if my dreams never met with reality.

This semi-halcyon, or rather less troubled, of my days in primary school were drawing ineluctably to a close and we were all to face the fearsome p7 teacher, Tiger MacNab. She was truly a monster who seemed like she had stepped straight out of the Inquisition. She subjected children to repeated questioning, even when it was clear they did not know the answer. Eventually when she had had enough of this form of torture, she delivered sharp punches with her knuckles. If they did not remember their tables, she would ask them out to the front of the class and drag them by the hair in front of us, making the child recite the tables line-by-line after her. It was dreadful to watch. And it was children who were slow learners who were her favourite victims. Many a child's confidence was shattered for ever by this abuse. And the parents turned a blind eye to it. She got results, or so they said. So keen were parents to get their children through the 11+ that nobody would rock the boat and object to any method presented to them as necessary. However it is my belief that her abuse did not improve anyone's performance by one mark. It caused such nervousness in all of us that we all probably underperformed. Certainly such tyranny dashed our trust in humanity to smithereens.

The day of the 11+ came. My father had been making me sit down at the dining-room table with sample I. Q. tests he got from my Auntie Millicent who taught in London and had access to papers. But they were for children a bit older than myself and I found them very hard to do. I resorted to cheating by looking up the answers at the back of the test-book. I was just too nervous to try to complete the test within the time allotted and I had to ensure that I got a higher score than Raymond, the banker's son, against whom my father had pitted me. So of course I was really nervous at the real event and do not think I did very well. But my poor friend, Jean, turned two pages in her IQ test and finished early. I tried in vain to signal to her. She got put in a C-stream, though undoubtedly a talented girl. In the secondary school after year 1, her teacher asked for her to be moved up to B-stream but Mr Stone, our headmaster, refused on the grounds that "she was only a railwayman's daughter."

I somehow got through though I got the impression from a remark of my father's that I had only just scraped through. And from then on, success in my school work, previously of little concern to me, became my number one mission. With the departure of Robbie and Billy, I had no friends nearby and the pressure to do well at school was immense, both from school and from my parents. I thus began to be very nervous around exam time even though I started to do really well at school and was always suddenly first in all my classes except Art where I was third.

All of my schoolmates were under similar pressure and we embarked on the next phase of our segregated lives in academic streams with superior toilets and facilities for the 'academic' children. This set up a dynamic where the C-girls hated the A girls and the B girls hated us both. My friends were thus from the A and B streams but I tried to keep up a friendship with Jean. This was doomed. She was always in different classes from me. She was keen to learn French and I tried to teach her at play-time, sitting together on a log-pile in the playground. And our friendship fizzled out. I am not sure if that was due to my being pre-occupied elsewhere and Jean's family left shortly after second year. I had truly liked Jean and felt terribly guilty about her plight. But one thing she was spared and that was the years of endless drudgery and meaningless hours of homework. Childhood really ended there for me.

And it was in my second year at secondary school that I nearly did lose my life. A healthy child till age seven, I then became prone to repeated throat infections and was dosed, as was the custom then, with antibiotics. But nothing serious. Then my mother nearly died from viral meningitis. I do not remember registering much about that. I felt no disturbance in my father's demeanour. In fact I think he spent the time flirting with one of my mother's oldest friends who came to look after us. I only found out afterwards that my mother had had a brush with death.

Then I had an infected spot or cut on my forehead. It was very itchy and I scratched at it. It got worse. And I developed septicaemia. The infection did not respond to antibiotics and for several days I lay in my bed with a very high fever. Then one day I hear a muttered medical consultation going on outside my bedroom door. I heard the doctor saying "We have to get her in to Aberdeen right now." My father came in the ambulance but I cannot remember much in the way of support from him. I believe he was crying and asking the ambulance staff whether I was going to die.

I was too ill to feel anything and was pretty soon unconscious for several days, coming round periodically for a few minutes as I was force-fed medicine which I vomited up. Nothing worked then I was injected with antibiotics and suddenly something worked. I came to groaning in pain one morning. An exasperated nurse spat at me "What are you groaning for? You have kept me awake all night." Welcome back to life for me.

As hard as it was at home, I found the week in hospital horrible. The food was appalling, I was in a room by myself and next door were a couple of little boys. One would howl in pain regularly every day as his dressings were changed by a gruff nurse. Nobody came to speak to me about my condition. One day I was wheeled briskly along a dark corridor to check by x-ray that I had no brain damage. Again no explanation. I had only a couple of parental visits and was grateful to get some comics from a girl who hated me but whose mother had, I suspected, obliged her to send them to me. Then one day the young handsome Church of Scotland minister pushed the door open. I was horrified, smitten with shyness especially as my face was still all swollen. He asked me if would like him to say a prayer for me. To be polite I said yes and that also meant I did not have to squirm to try to answer his concerned questions. From his sombre prayers I concluded that I must be dying.

However a few days later I was sent off home and spent a further three weeks off school. I was terribly thin and was told I had been very near death, touch and go. I remember actually feeling no pain only a tremendous peace and deep slumber. The teachers thought I would be really behind but I did one hour's school-work every day and was still top of the class -

which shows how inefficient it is to keep children at school for long hours.

The arena school did offer myself and some of my friends, however, was one on which we could displace our home distress. However fear-inspiring some of these professional characters in our lives were, our teachers became the target for our subversive anger. We used to hide behind bushes and scream insults at our Latin teacher as she laboured on her bike up the brae to school. We would make horrible noises with gay abandon in the English class as our teacher was stone deaf. One of our bolder members recited "Baa baa black sheep" instead of Grey's Elegy and got away with it. We even put bubble gum on teacher's chairs before class and threw a banger after our Latin teacher.

Occasionally such exploits earned us a real row but in general I think we were considered a class that was more interesting because we were more spirited. I suspect some of our teachers were not at all surprised that we needed to let off steam, given the tyranny of the school regime. They maybe even harboured sympathy for us knowing however that they still had to bring in exam results that honoured the school and promoted their own careers. Looking back, I think I was probably, if not the ring-leader, certainly a prime mover in these minor acts of insubordination. I was indeed viewed as a trouble-maker by my teachers. As I did well academically however my conduct at school never did prompt school concern or questions about my home-life.

When I was thirteen, my granddad died. I had been dimly aware that he was ill as he had a big bandage around his neck and there were dark remarks about him having throat cancer. This meant nothing to me as I did not know what cancer could do. When he did die, my mother and grandmother did not seem to be at all affected. My grandma came up to stay with us more often and spent Christmas and her birthdays with us from then on.

My mother later on in life told me that her father had been a wonderful father when she was a child but the sad reality is that he started drinking heavily when she was seven after her brother died. And by the time I came along this man was really scary. My grandma barked him out of his lair for mealtimes. He hobbled in to eat with us, leaning heavily all his massive weight on a shepherds crook, he was dressed in baggy brown plus fours, always wore a greasy bonnet and a heavy scowl. He said not a word during the meal. We kids all ate in silence, trying with all our might not to have a fit of giggles which would have earned us a   fearsome snarl from him and a rebuke from my grandma.

Thus it was quite understandable that his death meant nothing to me except that now we could venture into the room he had occupied to play and look through a set of binoculars kept there. We could chat freely at table. I sometimes wish I had known this man before he was wrecked by alcoholism. His nephew also told me years later he was a lovely man, which I found impossible to believe.

One tale that was told of him was that, during the war, when he had served in the Home Guard, he had been so drunk when coming home down the cliff path towards Craig Darroch bridge that he fell many feet down into the river and was washed up insensible on the Rhonay Isle. Not a family saga to sit proudly in any family annals. So much for guarding the home.

So all in all there was not one single man in my close childhood life who was not very damaged, damaging and scary. Not a good recipe for me to embark on the next chapter of my life – the years of my initiation into boys and teenage romance.

CHAPTER 3

Teenage Trials

Well, from fourteen on things started to really get 'intense' with a full academic programme which apparently needed us to do three to four hours homework every night, troubles at home and trying to navigate dealings with the other sex. I had no time to feel or reflect on my life. And in a way that suited my need to avoid the very painful emptiness that I tried to keep at bay. These gnawing feelings fuelled my drive to do well academically, which I did. However this earned me the envy of my peers and I had to compensate and become badly behaved in order to try to belong.

By modern standards my misconducts were pretty minor but I did draw an angry remark from my English teacher in my fourth year - "I advise you to go and see a doctor" – well, he was right, I did need help but when I did present for help a couple of years later with what should have been spotted as anorexia, I did not get it. But I am leaping ahead of myself.

I desperately tried to fit in at school and I did have a group of girl friends who were all in the A-stream. The B and C girls hated us and would not talk to us. We were a vital crew and lively but all in our different ways distressed and it came out not only in insubordination to our teachers and feuds with the non-academic girls and the stuck-up well-behaved older academic girls, but in perpetual in-fighting between us all. I had by this time developed a winsome and placating style with all so I was probably one girl who was never too badly ganged-up on. But even so, there was continual insecurity and back-biting between us, minor acts like emptying out each other's schoolbags, saying nasty things behind each others' backs, all the usual trials of girls trying to sort out their place in a world where we were prized now, not only academically, but also by how we looked. This was the age of the dirndle skirt, the hula hoop, then in my fourth year, the Beatles. We back-combed our hair, tried to shorten our skirts and tighten our trousers in the teeth of the cold stares of the Calvinist village elders.

None of my efforts in this fashion-department bore fruit at school as, although getting on well enough with girls, boys seemed to ignore me. I was rarely spoken to by a boy. I think I was the most ignored girl (apart from poor little Jessie who was multiply afflicted with buck teeth, cross eyes, ghastly pink NHS specs, the lot) and it profoundly affected my self-image as I grew up. My incredible shyness froze my tongue in attempting to even talk to boys and something about my manner must have put them off. There was also the fact that, because I did well at exams, I had a reputation as a swot. It was also well known that I had a scary father policing my social life.

In fact he used to follow myself and Elizabeth in his car and order us to get in. Once we revolted. He said his policing us was not of his own volition but was driven by our mother's insistence that we did not go around with 'undesirables.' But on the only occasion I managed to attract a date who should have been more than acceptable to my parents, my father showed just how much he wanted to control my interactions with boys. Jack Weston, the dux of a nearby school and thus one might consider a suitable friend for their daughter, took me to the cinema in Elgin. However the film ended too late for me to catch the bus. I had to ring Dad and ask him to come and collect me. As the car drew up, I was leaning against Elgin clock tower with Jack kissing me. Dad glowered at us. I said good night to Jack and got hastily into the car. Dad drove off fast but not before yelling at me "You bitch." My face smarted. He may have hit me - I cannot remember but my face and whole upper body burnt with humiliation. Jack never contacted me again after that. I had really really liked him and had I had a 'normal' father, my life might have been so different from that point on.

The men from whom my father should have protected his daughters were in fact his own drunken and sleazy friends. On their many visits to our home they made lecherous remarks, commenting on Elizabeth's legs and the like. My father even said to one of his cronies about a six-year old Elizabeth, asleep in her bed - "Are you not going up to kiss your girl-friend goodnight."

However the father-factor did not dent the popularity with boys of two of my sisters so again I thought my being spurned by them was all down to my being ugly. In fact I was not at all ugly but must have felt so inside.

Bleeding was pronounced a curse by my mother and we had to smuggle our soiled towels down to the boiler in the kitchen without being seen. The girls-cloakroom at school was the size of a cupboard and as I bled very heavily, I often used to go through several sanitary towels in one day. My legs would be raw with chafing if the tiny toilet-bucket was full and I could not change my sodden towel. I thus felt as if everyone could smell me and that did not help my self-confidence. Nearly every other girl apart from me had a boyfriend at some stage in secondary school and I could only conclude that I was very unlovable and unattractive, in spite of my care with my clothes and hair.

But the backdrop to all these teenage trials was the slow collapse of our family, as evidenced by the increasing plight of Rose. Always an emotionally expressive child, embarrassing me with joyous singing as we walked the road to school, and given to outbursts of laughter and tears in fast sequence, as a teenager her mood darkened, she wept a lot and lamented loudly to all at school and at home how she was hopeless at everything. The fact was that she was a good all-round student, she had however failed the 11-plus, and was placed in a B-stream because my father appealed on her behalf. But she really could not cope with the academic demands of Maths and Arithmetic. Many a night I would come in from playing and find her miserable, stuck with some problem. Sometimes she would be weeping over it. And sometime I, as her younger sister, could help her, not an easy position for either of us.

She began to be very religious and also to save her pocket money in a box labelled for the League of Pity (for destitute children.) Her earlier revolts ceased and she became seriously depressed. She had been the fourteen year-old who had dared to climb out of our bedroom window which had openings at either end. On many a night, she would walk along the narrow ledge at one end and clamber in at the other. This risk-taking stopped when she was sighted by a neighbour. But until my parents were then informed, Rose forbade me to tell on her – all I could do was watch with bated breath, aware that if she fell, she could be seriously injured or killed on the paving below.

Now she was not up for such acts of daring. She became cowed and fearful. And when I was fourteen, she left school and went to a Commercial College in Glasgow. It was clear that my father regarded such a daughter as a dud. And she did not even manage that. By the end of the first term the college sent her home saying she had problems. Much of it may have been down to the fact that she could not master shorthand and, given that she had the same problems with reading music and with maths, she may have had some form of dyslexia. Given the little regard my father felt for her career, her failure at it must have been the final nail in her coffin. From then on, she went downhill in a slow and agonized descent that took all of three years. She was packed off to mental hospital in Aberdeen at the age of sixteen. We were told not to tell anyone. This served to make me feel ashamed of her, myself and my family.

Her treatment I found out years later was the standard one dished out to emotionally troubled teenage girls at that time. Drugs and more drugs, insulin-induced comas, ECT and hours of knitting. She was with much older patients and she deteriorated. I remember finding it a relief when she was away from home because it was horrible to live with. Sometimes she had big cuts down her arms. We were instructed not to refer to them or enquire about them, though on one occasion my mother told me, implausibly, the wounds were caused by falling into the green house. Another time Rose had a huge red raw surgical scar down her stomach. I was not told why. So I could only assume that she had had an abortion, though the scar was actually vertically down. I found out years later it was caused by the fact she had swallowed a fork and had to be cut open in an emergency procedure.

She slept in the same bedroom, sometimes the same bed, as myself. Being close to such wounds and her upset in those years made me feel full of very intense mixed feelings. One was of care, where I would go upstairs to see her after school and try to cheer her up with daft stories I concocted about our teachers. She would be lying in bed drugged. I would try to reassure her about her capacities. I would listen to her. But I also felt terribly embarrassed by her residence in the 'nut-house' and ashamed of her and her state. Her non-stop laments irked me. And they clearly drove my mother mad. Once Rose was whining on about how useless she was and my mother hit her hard on the head with the hoover end. She burst into tears and went home with Joan, a friend of ours who had witnessed my mother in action. Joan's parents were shocked. So used was I to our family ways that I felt nothing, even thinking that Rose should not have gone on like that and what did she deserve but to get hit.

Dad responded to Rose's state by taking to his bed as often as he could, moaning, and praising me for trying to cheer Rose up. "Keep up the good work" - he said he could not deal with it. Somehow he expected his fourteen-year old daughter to deal with his share of showing care. My mother also charged me with cheering him up as well. I did not at all like giving energy to a man who terrorised us and then acted pathetic.

I think I really felt totally powerless and frozen. One day I came home and went upstairs as usual to see Rose. This time she was lying on the floor, drugged and floppy, and her hands were all bloodied. She had climbed out of bed and broken one of my mother's precious ornaments. It lay smashed beside her. Then she had slumped down and was crying over the shards. She had cut herself badly, possibly deliberately. I screamed for our mother. She rushed in and I feared she would hit Rose again. But I was trying to drag Rose to her feet and my mother and I then put her in bed. But next day she had gone, back to the loony bin.

So it went on from year to year and I was going to school as normal, acting like a normal school-girl and trying to be an academic and social success.

It came as no shock to me when she finally, at the age of nineteen, hanged herself in hospital. It was Easter. Thirty years later I learnt that Dad had gone into Aberdeen with Mum and they had taken Rose out for a trip to the beach. Dad had asked Rose if she wanted to come home for the holiday. She said no. And then told him she was frightened of him. He started to cry and so did she.

Then next day I became somehow aware of some difficult phone call. I went and stood at the top of the stairs looking down on my father's head. I heard him gasping. It was just after lunch. He said "Oh no" and then put the phone down and went fast into the living room. I went down and he said that Rose had died.

Everyone was there and very quiet. I asked him how, he said the poor little thing had died of convulsions. I did not believe him. I felt angry at him for covering things up. It took me twelve years to find out the bare facts and it was not from my family. It came from a member of medical staff treating me for trauma.

I sat down at a table by a window below which the river Spey flowed as beautiful as ever. All of us were gathered in silence in the living room. Only Ewan shed a few tears. He told me years later that he felt he ought to. Nobody said anything for a long time. Then I said "Can I still go to the dance this evening?" Dad said "No, of course you cannot go. It is not at all suitable when you sister has just died." "Why not?" I demanded. "It would seem heartless" he replied. I felt a surge of rage. Why did Rose spoil everything for me so much? No doubt my desire was really for life to go on as normal.

And the pain had long before gone underground, too hard to handle. But the sheer force it took to keep it in subterranean terrain propelled my life into repeated re-enactments of loss and drew me over and over to violent people. It also, years later, fuelled terrible volcanic eruptions at partners who later stood in for my parents. These brought with them unspeakable self-loathing, as I was then completely unable to stem the flow of delayed shock and trauma, sometimes even when my children were present. I had sworn to myself I would never subject my children to the terrible parental fights that had scarred my childhood. It took me over ten years to visit the grave which appeared some years later.

On the day of her death, however, all I note in my diary was "Rose died today" then I listed the dates for my upcoming Higher exams which would determine whether I got into university or not. I felt total panic, but not about the tragic death, only about whether I would make the academic grade.

Nobody spoke to me about Rose's death except one of my friends who hesitantly said she was very sorry. I replied stoically that it was probably for the best, she was suffering terribly. One of the teachers was slightly delicate with me on my first day back at school, reserving his bark for all the others in my class, but not me.

There was no visible sign of mourning in the family. After the funeral a silence on the subject descended like a black pall. However, when the dog died three weeks after Rose's death, I came into the kitchen to find Mum on the floor sobbing inconsolably as she clutched the dead body. I felt a brief flash of rage. In my head were the words "Well, you can cry over the dog but not over your daughter." Dad did once try to speak to me about it. I was stuck up in the attic frantically immersing myself in studying. He came up the ladder in tears and said he wanted to talk to me about Rose. I rasped "Go away. You will make me fail my exams." I did not want to talk about it to him at all, nor did I want to be used by my father as his support.

He and my mother were locked in yet further combat – this time over my father's claim that, had my mother allowed Rose to stay at home more, she would not have got so ill. Dad lashed out a lot in the first few days of shock as he tried no doubt to displace his own guilt onto others, including the hospital for placing his daughter that last night in a high-security ward with lot of older and very disturbed patients.

After one of these heated rows Mum retreated up to their bedroom and shut the door. A few hours later, Dad asked me to get Mum down for tea. I knocked on the door and told her tea was ready. No response. I tried the door-handle – it was locked. My heart tightened in fear. I raised my voice and asked my mum if she was alright. After a continuation of the silence through several of my pleas, I got frantic and started throwing myself against the door in sheer terror that she also had taken her own life.

Still no response through an agony of desperate waiting. Then a harsh utterance swamped me with relief but its content hacked my soul to shreds. "Go away." "Go away. You are all more trouble than you are worth. I wish you had never been born." I collapsed into the twelve-year old arms of poor Ewan who had been standing stock-still beside me with an ashen face. My father appeared and summoned us to eat - no subsequent words of comfort from him and no subsequent words of apology or comfort from my mother.

Understandably I was completely unable to deal with my feelings and proceeded instead to sail through my exams, gaining five A-passes at one sitting, remarkably rare at that time. I got through the summer holidays and being considered too young to go to university, my friend Gillian and I stayed on to do sixth year and sit a bursary competition. My father wanted me to try for Oxbridge but I refused - I think I felt the pressure was too great - but I consented to my father's opinion that I should go to St Andrew's, being totally politically naïve and unaware that it was an upper-class enclave of mainly Oxbridge rejects.

My sixth year proved to be nothing other than marking time. None of the class-teachers had space in their timetables to tutor Gillian and I and we had to sit in the back of each class and get on with preparing ourselves for the bursary work with very little input. One of my tasks was to study Spenser's Fairie Queen and the rest of the reading was also completely equally alienating. I did try for over six months then early in the spring, I remember being at the fireside with Ewan and Mum. I suddenly realized that I could not go on. I flung the Faerie Queen volume to the floor, blurting out that I was going to leave school. And this I did. I got a job waitressing in the Palace Hotel in Grantown which served mainly wealthy visitors up for fishing. I lived in the hotel during the week and came home at the weekends.

I knew nobody in Grantown, there was an obnoxious slightly older male student in a gap-year also on the staff, a horrible head waitress who terrified me and a drunken older waiter. So from one bad situation to another but at this stage in my life I had no capacity to register, let alone express, my bleak feelings. What did happen however was that I began to restrict my eating but failed miserably in the making-myself-sick department. Within a few months I became very thin and my periods stopped. I mentioned this to mum who took me to the doctors. He asked me a few curt questions, prodded me in the tummy, presumably suspecting that I was pregnant, asked me nothing relevant about eating or possible grief and sent me home to continue untreated.

This problem changed when I set off in the autumn for my first term at St Andrews. This was a very traditional university and we had to wear red academic gowns and were expected to live in supervised halls of residence for our first year, and thereafter too. We were basically in loco parentis, having to sign in at night by eleven if we had been out. The meals however were wonderful and there was also a huge afternoon tea at four. I threw myself into my studies and also into over-eating. This somehow did not result in overweight so never showed up as a problem, though I was grimly aware that gorging to the stage of sickness was shameful and meant something was wrong with me.

I made friends with three other Scottish girls and soon found out that students fell into two distinct classes, debs and plebs. I was not really even a pleb – plebs all seemed to know each other from big city–schools and I did not meet any other Scottish student who came from rural Scotland. My three Scottish friends were pleasant but fairly traditional and lacked the rebellious streak of my former circles. In my later University years, when I moved out of official accommodation, I had a different range of friends. In my final year I want back in to halls and was friendly with two other final year students, a couple called Jeff and Pamela, who were mathematicians and always falling out with each other.

I started off studying French and German but soon found myself at sea amidst a crowd of students from England or private schools who had done A- levels and at whom the course was pitched. It would not be so easy for me to shine as before in such a set-up so in my second year I switched and from then on landed up doing social sciences with my final degree in politics and economics. My choice was based on discovering that these were subjects I could get high marks in with the least effort. However it meant that in my last two years I was in small classes which consisted of myself and four young men with whom I competed. I was one of two of us who got firsts and I and the biggest swot in the universe shared joint class medals.

My romantic life was still struggling. I threw myself into trying to find a boy-friend, attended all the student dances I could but nobody wanted to 'go out' with me. The man I landed up most with was Benji, debauched and drunken son of some eminent academic who was brilliant and spent most of his time in an alcoholic daze but seemed to sail through his studies. He never asked me out. I relied on him picking me up in the last few minutes of the 'hops.' St Andrew's social life revolved around the holding every term of several balls at the various Halls of Residence and I managed to avoid nearly all of them except those where I lived. It was agony finding someone to partner me and agony to find a ball dress I felt at all good in. Benji came to one with me, distinguishing us as a couple by running around in a suit of armour he grabbed from the entrance. Then I mistakenly put my elbow through a window. The Hall Warden was highly displeased with me indeed. And I certainly did not enjoy it.

But I still persisted on my romantic quest on home-ground at the drunken dances held in the villages. Eventually I was fed up of being a virgin. Elizabeth had had a steady boyfriend by sixteen. So I 'did it' with a young steel erector called Sam who was working temporarily in Speyside. It was not a memorable night but it launched me on several years of casual sexual encounters which took me into all sorts of situations. If I liked the look of a boy, I went for him and that was how it went. Invariably my choices were often of very drunken young men who certainly never treated me like a girlfriend. And significantly enough I never expected them to - sex itself was enough to make me feel I mattered momentarily and became an aim in itself.

Such a life-style was not one I chose or had any control over but was the only way at the time that I seemed to be able to get attention. It was bound to lead to trouble. And it did.

CHAPTER 4

The Keys to the Door

On reaching our majority, we would suppose one writes the script of our life free from parental interference and equipped with all the tools of adulthood. Reading my diaries over the years following twenty-one does not fill me with pride. And I have to subscribe to the view that much of the adult life we live is run using very early childhood tapes at a deep unconscious level. Certainly my twenties were full of driven conduct which really sabotaged those years so key in setting off on the key-tasks of career and home-building.

I did get a good degree, investing a lot of nervous energy into this. A male tutor had kindly told me in my third year that I should stay on to do a full honours degree – I had been toying with the idea of leaving as I hated the milieu and my subjects. He said that I could pull myself up by the boot-straps. I was surprised and a bit insulted as it had never occurred to me that I was being experienced as coming from the nether classes. This would have caused great consternation for my snobbish mother. Anyway, not having the slightest idea what else to do with my life, I did stay on and I suppose I should be proud of the fact that I not only got a class-medal in both my fourth and fifth years but also that I got a first in economics. I was the only woman in my class and this was indeed a big success. But such was the misery in my emotional life and my low self-esteem that my academic success did not register at all on my well-being.

This was still dictated by my continuing difficulty in finding a decent boyfriend. In my fourth year, despairing of the men at St Andrew's, I went down to Edinburgh most weekends and hung out with Elizabeth's crowd, which included many old Watsonians who were really a drunken and empty lot. There was no communication from the men to women, just drinking and listening to men pounding away on guitars. But I felt honoured to become the girl-friend of one of the crew, Angus, a trainee silver-smith, the black sheep of his family, which included renowned surgeons and the like. Angus did excel in the amounts of alcohol he consumed.

I say he was my boy-friend but really he showed no signs of it. I hung out with the crowd and at the end of the evening, we fell into bed. We used contraceptives but somehow I became pregnant. Predictably Angus wanted me to get rid of it pronto. And in such a scenario I entertained no other possibility. Firstly Angus's brother, a medical student, secured some pills for me which were supposed to hopefully cause a miscarriage. But no such luck and I had to endure the humiliation of a visit to a psychiatrist in the nearby hospital in Leven and convince him that continuing with a pregnancy might endanger my health.

The law had just changed to allow abortions on these grounds but the doctor I saw made sure he made my interview an unpleasant experience. However I got an abortion on the NHS in the cottage hospital in St Andrews. I woke up sobbing. I told nobody at university but on my first day in the ward, I was surprised and embarrassed to have a male visitor, Ken, from my class. I did not ask how he knew but it also seems my room-mate in digs had also guessed. Ken brought me some grapes and was very kind - the only person who was. Elizabeth told me that I was a disgrace to the family. Then Angus dumped me, informing me that Elizabeth and her friend Fiona had had a talk with him and told him he was 'bad for me', thus he was doing me a service and ending it. Twenty five years later I confronted Elizabeth with this. But she angrily retorted that Angus had just tried to shift the blame on to her and Fiona. To this day I rather believe Angus to have told the truth - what he told me did chime with my experience of Elizabeth. But even so it was his choice to act as he did, whatever others said to him.

Certainly the end of that relationship was salutary, though I was really distraught at the time. I wrote Angus a couple of upset letters, especially when he informed me that his mother had burnt my best coat which I had left in one of his cupboards "because it smelled." Whatever his mother may or may not have said, he could have spared me that further humiliation.

I was also at that time seeing one of my lecturers, a Welsh working-class communist who had the gift of the gab. He was really worshipped by the student-body for his wit and learning. He was infatuated with me and wanted to marry me, even though I was pregnant with someone else's child. As he was twenty eight, he seemed like an old man to me and, though I went out with him for many months, at that time, love in my book equated to storms and cruelty and I could not return his feelings.

The summer after the abortion I was to spend in Edinburgh preparing for my final year. Elizabeth had been seeing this very handsome man called Kenneth for eighteen months or so and she told me she had finished with him. She set off to go fruit-picking in Lincoln, instructing him to make sure I was not lonely. Kenneth used to visit me in my bed-sit. I had always been dead attracted to him and envied the time he devoted to Elizabeth, often lying in bed with her for hours chatting.

Gradually it became clear that he was keen on me. We discussed the situation. He also assured me that he and Elizabeth were through and so we felt the way was open for us to start a relationship which went on for almost four years. It was the first time I was in love and had my love returned. Kenneth looked like Jim Morrison of the Doors, and with such a boy-friend, I felt that I had at last become equal to other women.

Sadly however Elizabeth went beserk, saying that she and Kenneth had not finished their relationship and she bore a grudge about me and her boyfriends for many years. Moreover I treated Dylan, my lecturer lover, very badly. We had still been going out in the summer and I could not bring myself to hurt him by telling him about Ken. I let Dylan travel all the way up from Wales to visit me with his best mate, only to find me ensconced with Kenneth. This must have really hurt and humiliated him and shows the extent of my inability to deal with basic emotional communication. For years I have tried unsuccessfully to contact Dylan to try to explain properly my dreadful conduct.

Apart from that, the following six months were one of the happiest periods of my life. Kenneth had attended Heriot's school in Edinburgh and had been educated well in literature. He introduced me to amazing authors I had never heard of, like Hess and Grass and also he had an exciting taste in music including Country Jo Mac Donald, Frank Zappa, the Doors, Captain Beefheart and the Love. We spent many happy hours together though Kenneth was terrified of getting me pregnant and generally could not cope with full-on sex.

When my university term resumed we visited each other at weekends. He was one year behind me, also doing economics but at Heriot Watt University. We often studied together and with Jeff as a friend also, in my final year, though horribly stressful, I felt some sort of security for the first and possibly only time in my life.

However when I moved to Edinburgh at the end of my degree to look for work, trouble started between us. I shared a series of flats or bedsits, was often very lonely and no longer had most of my energy invested in getting a good degree. I desperately wanted Kenneth to move in with me - he stubbornly refused. His father had died just after the war and his mother had struggled to raise him and his two sisters in a council house in Pilton. Kenneth said he did not want to leave his mother in the lurch. I pointed out that she still had his two older sisters at home and it became a horrible tug-of-war between us, with my venting rage so intensely that I realized I had a problem. I went for psychological help. This started my career in the psychiatric system.

Meanwhile my work-career started after a few months of unemployment in which I succumbed to a severe attack of broncho-pneumonia that left my chest permanently weakened. Those winter months before I got a job in the Scottish office as an Assistant Research Officer were very hard and this took a further toll on my relationship with Ken.

For a good few weeks I did not have my own accommodation and had to sleep in a makeshift bed on Elizabeth's floor in the flat she shared with four other girls. Two of them were very judgemental and felt nothing of telling me more than once that they would never sign on for unemployment benefit, they would take any old job. Elizabeth clearly found their attitude to me a problem for her and she was quite nasty to me about my needing to stay with her, even though I was so ill with coughing that I was in no fit state to look for a flat and move and I had little money to pay for rent. This also in spite of the fact that for two years I had given Elizabeth a large part of a bursary I had won to compensate for the fact that Dad did not give her the parental support contribution she was due.

The job I got was in the first few months terribly boring and demoralising as the Research Unit had expanded fast and had not really got work-projects set up for me and the other two new graduates. Many days there was nothing really for me to do and I felt unwanted and useless, now not only by Kenneth but also as a worker.

Then I was given a big project on pre-school planning and funding which I did so well that my work was commended by the Treasury. But these years were quite demanding because I worried about my performance and had occasionally to fly down to London and have meetings with posh English senior civil servants who were twenty years my senior. I was lucky however to have a really nice boss called Alistair and this helped but in general it just got too much holding down this job and dealing with the inner turmoil that started to get stirred up by my therapy. And so in 1973 I resigned at the age of twenty-seven. This was the end of my formal professional career using my degree and earning a good salary, much to my parent's disgust. They had no idea of what was really happening to me and what was behind my 'dropping-out'.

In fact the truth was that three years into the job and my career was becoming incompatible with my chaotic life-style. I was by this time about eighteen months into weekly therapy sessions at the Royal Edinburgh Psychiatric OP Unit. These sessions were with a CPN called Mrs Black who was kindly and insightful but very very conventional. She started helping me excavate my childhood, not the facts, of which I had an unusually excellent memory, but the feelings about which I felt numb. She urged me to visit Rose's grave, something I had known I did not want to do. There had not been a stone there for the first few years, nobody in the family mentioned it and I certainly did not want to see it. In fact the whole topic of Rose and her death was erased from family talk.

As we progressed into my feelings, my outer life became more distressed, my sleep became very disordered and so did my relationships with men. Kenneth had at first also gone for therapy at the unit and had been judged as needing it and bringing his own problems into our by-this-time troubled dynamic. This was a relief to me as I often was sure it was solely myself that was the problem as it was I who felt such turmoil about it and such dissatisfaction with his detachment. But after a few weeks, Kenneth stopped attending, saying he did not think he needed it. Sadly his further relationship breakdowns indicated that he did.

I meanwhile went from man to man, including, with no scruples, one of Kenny's friends and periodically I would dump him. I spent all my time out and about visiting people or having people round to my flat. I also attended the University film club regularly, often by myself. I had a wide circle of friends but none of them did I really let close, so although I lamented with them about my problems with Kenneth or how boring my job was, they never knew about the underlying reasons. But in fact by this time I was in a very fragile state emotionally and felt utterly alone and stricken with this.

Moreover I finally blew it with Kenny, taking up with a much younger and seriously disturbed addicted young man called Lincoln. He was of mixed race, came from Chelmsford in Essex and was one of 6 boys in a mixed marriage between a black Jamaican and a white working-class Yorkshire lass. Lincoln had been a model child but turned into a rebel in his early adolescence and ran away from home to London where he lived in the notorious 44a Piccadilly squat. He was introduced to drugs at the age of fourteen by someone he called Dr Nick who seemed to run the squat. Behind his flight from home was the fact that his father was very heavy-handed and scary.

Being from a rural backwater I was very naive in my understanding of drug issues and did not really have any idea of the nature or severity of Lincoln's addictions when we first joined up. And after messing him about a bit, then him repaying me in kind, I fell for him hook, line and sinker.

Needless to say, Mrs Black was appalled that I should be involved with such a 'sociopath' and even more so when she learnt that he had initiated me into LSD. I took it only once aged twenty-six and had such a mixed trip, with a full blown case of the horrors, that I steered clear of it for another eight years. I smoked dope a bit, drank with the crowd and swallowed Valium which was liberally prescribed to assist my sleep. This was before the days of knowledge of the addictive nature of this class of drugs but soon, to get even a few hours of sleep, I had to keep increasing the dose. Then I was given a stronger drug, then another class, until eventually I was swallowing Sodium Amytal and Tuinal in quantities but they also had eventually little effect on my ability to sleep. I was desperate.

My relationship with Lincoln was fraught with furious rows in which he often gave me kickings, threw me down stairs, or started to throttle me. But all I was afraid of was that he would leave me. Clearly this world of addiction, violence and chaos was not compatible with the stability I needed for the demands of working as a professional career civil-servant and I chose the non-career path.

Thus what I did was line up a trip to the USA on a Churchill fellowship to study compensatory programmes there for pre-school children. This was for three months – all expenses paid. One of the factors behind my finally ending things with Kenny was that, when I had raised the subject of this trip with him, he told me I should take it. I was mad at him as I wanted him to say that he would really miss me and did not want me to go. But no such response. Lincoln however cut up really rough about my plans. But off I went.

I had a good subsistence rate and prepared a detailed itinerary. But really I was quite unfit for such a trip with such a reliance on Valium to get by and knowing nobody in the USA. I had also for over a year been experiencing   night-time horrors or flash-backs with heavy religious symbology, probably induced by the prescribed medication. In the few hours I managed to sleep I was often in a realm I can only describe as hell.

But I did my fellowship, suffering terrible terror and loneliness and not really knowing how to find my feet in such a different culture whilst travelling from place to place. I teamed up for a couple of weeks with a lovely young French student, who was doing business-studies and was enamoured of the American dream, but we had different itineraries and at this point, my emotional numbing put me into a very dangerous arena.

I had been hanging out with some young black guys in the YMCA where I lived in the heart of Manhattan at 34th street. I was blind to the fact that most of these guys were Vietnam vets on drug rehab programmes - they were smartly dressed, seemed well-spoken and they told me that they were psychologists and the like. And I certainly found many of them strongly attractive.

One day I was to visit a young woman puppeteer whom I had met at one of the pre-school centres. I set off across the centre of Manhattan, meeting with a black veteran whom I had been introduced to a few days before. He was called Washington. He asked me where I was off to and offered to accompany me as he said I would have to cross some dangerous parts of the city. I trustingly accepted his offer and when we come to the hotel he was staying in and he said he wanted to nip up to his room to collect his jacket, I accepted his invitation to pop up with him without a second's thought.

However when we reached the twenty-first floor and walked down a long corridor, as he stopped to open his door, I suddenly felt the hackles on my head stand up. Too late. He quickly opened the door, grabbed me and shoved me into a small dark room. He seized the bottle of wine I was carrying to my friend's, smashed it and held the broken end up to my throat. He demanded to have sex. I stood there, rooted to the spot and said nothing. He then hurled me to the window and pushed my head out. He told me if I did not have sex with him he would throw me out and that he had thrown another woman out just recently. Clearly this was not very convincing as such a crime would not have gone without repercussions but I knew that this man was too volatile to muck about with and I acquiesced to sex. I started to act placatingly to him.

Afterwards he went all pathetic, crying and wanting me to be his girl-friend. However, again suddenly, he jumped up out of bed and started acting crazy once more. He took my bag into his bathroom and shortly after came out and gave it back to me. Clearly he had robbed me but I was not going to quibble. I knew I had to keep him calm to get out. And that is what I did. I found my way to my friend's and told her. She was horrified. She recommended I get some counselling.

So when I got back to the YMCA I made an urgent appointment with a resident counsellor. When he found out that my rapist was black his attitude to me became punitive – "What do you expect" he said "if you knock about with niggers?"

I left New York shortly after as my schedule required me to travel south. My sleep deteriorated. My Valium intake increased and at one point I was getting the 'horrors' visually in daylight hours, probably due to erratic use of Valium. I spent the next few weeks in the USA trying to keep to my schedule and having sex with a further two guys en route. I cannot remember now exactly what the sequence of events was during that awful time but at some stage I realized I was pregnant. I was not certain who the father of the child might be, I did not think it was Lincoln's or the young Frenchman's but I could not be sure. My other three possibilities were the rapist's, and my one-night stands, travelling businessmen. I knew I should go straight back to Edinburgh.

I got there just before Christmas and my first job was to fix up abortion number two. A lovely friend from school, Diana, let me sleep in a little room in the flat she lived in with her husband, Nigel, and little boy, Stephen.

In those next few weeks my health deteriorated. I had the second abortion and felt utterly lost. This was not helped by the matron in charge of the gynie ward who insisted on asking me publicly why I had had an abortion. I knew she had read my file. I did not want to say the word 'rape' out loud in the open ward in which

I was in bed bleeding away the last of the pregnancy and feeling very wobbly. So I said "I do not feel responsible enough to look after a baby" to which she retorted "You were responsible enough to conceive it." All this to the background accompaniment of weeping by a young woman who had just had a miscarriage.

I told nobody about the rape though I did tell a couple of women friends in the research team that I was to have an abortion and they were quite supportive. It goes without saying that I told nobody in my family and in particular not Elizabeth after her judging me over abortion number one.

I went to see Mrs Black, hoping for some ongoing support. She told me "Oh dear, this is what we thought would happen if you went to New York" - we being herself and my GP. I wondered angrily why in that case they had not advised me to postpone my trip. I however continued to see her and eventually, after much coaxing from her, went to visit Rose's grave for the first time. The night before, I had one of the worst waking dreams ever, with a little black incubus exiting my body and scrabbling around the floor. I felt very little when I saw the grave except a surge of anger at the inscription on it "Safe in the arms of Jesus." I thought angrily "Not so."

I returned to Edinburgh, only to be told, at this point of highest need in my therapy, that Mrs Black was to be transferred and that I could not get any more therapy at the Royal Ed.

It was winter and Lincoln had come back up to Edinburgh and reconnected with me. I moved out from Diana's where I had had much kindness but was also disturbed by their stormy relationship. Then I decided to go down south to purportedly write up my fellowship and pick up with Lincoln. I met up with him in London and he was desperate to have a child, completely unrealistically since he was still not even twenty and had no training, job or desire to earn a living. He had also moved about so much he had problems signing on. But given my fragile state, my infatuation with him and my desperate need to replace the recently aborted child, this seemed the thing that would help give my life a meaning.

I got pregnant straightaway, moved to Cambridge and lived camping for a few weeks with friends then moved into a room with a couple who took in tenants. I had one room there. Lincoln came to live with me. But with myself in a very distraught state and him with no job or money, I was continually rowing with him. When I was about four months pregnant he walked out.

I was relieved. The next few months I tried my best to get by. My new doctor referred me to group psychotherapy at Addenbrokes and I was told by a psychiatrist that I was seriously ill and should go back to Edinburgh for one-to-one therapy. I knew however that that was not now available for me in Edinburgh. I stayed on in Cambridge trying to cope. I wrote up my fellowship in a basic way. I also tried to prepare for the birth of my child. I had only two friends in town, Fiona and Greg, but there were problems there as Greg fell for me and Fiona started threatening suicide if I 'stole' Greg away. I was quite drawn to Greg who wanted to be with me and be father to the baby but with someone threatening suicide, there was no way I could or would act to further my own interests.

There were two situations at that time which illustrate just what a plight I was in. One was where Greg and Fiona took me out to visit some American friends of Greg's from the nearby air-base. They were all high on drugs and some of them had motor-bikes on which they speeded about whilst very drugged. One asked me if I wanted a ride on the back with him. Without any hesitation I jumped astride and we set off. He rocketed up to eighty m.p.h. with my hanging on urging him on.

The other dreadful story is when a friend of Greg's needed a partner for a May ball. He was an upper-class twit whom I did not know. So I was asked to be his escort. I met up with him at the ball - I was very surprised to see a handsome young man before me and asked myself why he had not been able find himself a partner. But he ignored me all night. I just stood, sat or walked about by myself amidst crowds of merry-makers. I had gone to some trouble to pretty myself up for the occasion, a Cambridge May ball, my goodness. And I was painfully aware that he knew that I knew only Fiona and Greg there. However they also left me very much to get on with things. I felt I could not approach them.

When I had raised queries with Fiona about attending the ball with a man on whom I had never even clapped eyes, I was pressurised by her. She had been trying to find this man a partner. She told me that I should be grateful to get an opportunity to attend such a prestigious event. Instead of going home after half an hour of neglect, I hung on by myself all evening on the edge of the groups of gay revellers, pretending to be enjoying myself. In fact understandably I felt totally spare and humiliated. I cannot remember if he escorted me home. I seem to remember walking back by myself at about two a.m. under a starry sky. I cannot imagine what I felt as I walked. I think I expected nothing better for myself and had no idea how to walk away earlier from such a humiliating experience.

Next I moved again into digs with a single mother with two little boys. I had a tiny cell of a freezing bedroom. I could not sleep. The single mum was a very messed up working-class woman with a foul attitude to her kids.

I decided I should move back to Edinburgh after the baby was born in November. So in the summer of 1974, I visited Edinburgh and, with the help of a good solicitor recommended by my friend Jan, I found a small but sound flat in Holyrood, in a tenement and on the fourth floor, not so easy, it turned out, for a lone mother, a baby and shopping.

Then I went back to Cambridge to finish writing up my fellowship and prepare for the birth of my baby.

CHAPTER 5

Nest Building

The last few months of pregnancy dragged by as they do for most expectant mothers. I was superficially in o.k health at the physical level with the development of varicose veins my only bother. But my emotional and psychological state was dire. Immediately I found out I was pregnant, I at once stopped taking any major tranquillizers and relied on Valium for a precious few hours of sleep. I tried to ration it and nights were sheer hell lying awake, hour after hour, in an agony of nameless dread. When I did sleep I often had horrific flash-backs. I had no friends in this divided town apart from Fiona and Greg but the difficult dynamic between us three persisted.

I cannot remember whom in the family I told about the pregnancy, though Elizabeth did know and came to Cambridge twice in the summer, once to see Fiona and myself and then to accompany me to London for the presentation by Prince Charles of a medallion for my fellowship. Then one time she came, Lincoln was there and we went punting on a sunny spring day. I intuited she had told my parents but I heard nothing from them or from my other siblings. But in a way, this did not impact on me as by this time I suppose I had written my family off. I attended group psycho-therapy and made trips to the shops and the library but that was my life.

Luckily I was also given the support of a CPN at this stage and I visited her office once a week. She was a lovely young American who was like a breath of fresh air and seemed to genuinely care for me, the only person in my life at that time who seemed to.

When I was about eight months pregnant, I got a letter from Lincoln saying he had sorted himself out now and wanted to take responsibility for me and the baby. He planned to come and see me. I replied asking him not to. I was suspicious that he had only approached me for a place for the winter. I also believed it was hard enough for me to cope with my trauma and depression as it was, without the stress of the instability his being with me would, I thought, entail. I could not see him changing his life-style and was clear I did not want any child of mine to be around the conflict that had so marred my childhood. He came anyway and my landlady went to the door. When I followed and said it was '*him*' she snarled "Go away – Gale does not want you." He turned on his heel and walked away and that was that for a good year or so.

Then things got really horrible for me in my digs as my landlady had gone into my cell of a bed-room and informed me it was too untidy. I was really floored and mentioned this to my CPN. She visited my digs and on seeing the room and getting a flavour of the atmosphere determined she would get me out of there. So the last few weeks of my pregnancy were spent in a lovely big room in a Vicarage in the outskirts of Cambridge at Cherry Hinton, the home of a pleasant upper-class family headed by the Rev Jones.

They had five children, four of whom were away at boarding school which accounted for their being able to offer me a home at this time. Their last child, Elsie, was about one and had been born with Downes

Syndrome. The idea was that now and again I could be in the house when Mrs Jones had to go out. But I do not remember spending any time looking after Elsie. I ate with the family, which I found hard as the Rev was very formal and emotionally distant, though he really tried to be kind to me.

At last I was at my due date but went over it by two weeks and was informed that I had to go into Addenbrokes Hospital on November 22nd for an induction. It had not even crossed my mind that anyone of my family would care enough to be there for me and in fact the weekend of the 22nd just happened to be the date set for the wedding of my brother, Ewan. There could be no contest between that and my delivering of a mixed race, illegitimate baby. Nobody of my family mentioned supporting me in any way. But my landlady, Mrs Jones, offered to be there for me and though I was sort of glad, I was also a bit embarrassed.   I felt I could not refuse as it would hurt her feelings and she was dead keen to attend, never having been at a birth.

It was a trial of a labour as most inductions are. I do not remember much about it except that at the end, Mrs Jones was encouraging me. Megan was born about ten at night and I was so exhausted from the hormones and drugs that I lost consciousness without seeing my daughter. It was eight hours later at six in the morning that the nurses brought me to her. They were really kind and assured me that they had never seen such a beautiful baby. And truly she was enchanting, just perfect. I bonded straight away, in spite of feeling dreadfully ill.

I think Greg and Fiona visited me but nobody else and I returned to the vicarage for a month before my room would be needed by the children and just before Christmas I took Megan up to Edinburgh in the train. My own flat would not be vacant for a few months but a friend had lent me his flat whilst he went to his family. I arrived on a freezing night just before Christmas and, as I was leaving the taxi and carrying Megan into the flat, someone made off with one of my suitcases, which I had had to leave on the pavement. It had a lot of our clothes in it. Luckily the other case had enough for our stay but the   first Christmas I had with Megan we spent alone. However my mother broke her silence and rang me. Moreover I had the flu but my focus on my baby helped me endure such a lonely festive period.

I set off back to Cambridge for a few weeks until my flat should be vacant. Elizabeth visited, I had a Christening for Megan. Greg and Fiona were delighted to be god-parents. As the minister poured the consecrated water over her tiny head, Megan tilted her face towards me and her beautiful features became illuminated for a brief moment. It was one of my first moments of numinousness.

The time passed somehow with a lovely weekend at the Cambridge folk festival with Fiona and Greg then a wonderful friend, Arthur, who had been in fact my dentist, came and drove me, Megan and a lot of my remaining belongings back to Edinburgh to our new home.

It was a cosy two-room flat with a cupboard-kitchen and tiny bathroom. I managed to get all the furniture I needed and set about getting curtains and sanding

Megan's floor. About the curtains there was a nasty episode as Greg gave me a set of lovely curtains from his parent's house. Then his mother saw a photo of Megan and decided she was Greg's child. Greg had often described his mother's neurosis before but it was very painful and embarrassing to be on the receiving end of it – he reported her as saying she would not give one penny to her son's bastard child!! Straightaway in anger she demanded he bring the curtains back – awful for him and also for Fiona who did not utter a word about the whole scenario. Did she also think that Greg had fathered Megan? – I will never know.

In spite of such initial setbacks I carried on steadfastly from day to day building a new life for me and Megan as a family. I still felt very ill much of the time and my sleep was really awful. I suffered a lot from dreadful loneliness and social isolation. I still had to stay on various drugs to get by and I had a social worker for support. I gather that they eventually reported that I was a remarkable and caring mother. I doted on Megan, read to her, played with her and she was my top priority.

Meanwhile not a word from my family until Megan was about six months old and my mother decided she could brave a visit. I think Elizabeth had assured her that the baby did not look like a little black Sambo. Anyway my mother adored Megan and was good to her from that time on. And Megan grew to be very close to her and eventually to my father. From then on, I took her back to the family home at Christmas and usually in the summer.

I started to make friends. As it happened my friend, Catherine, had just had a baby, Astrid, a couple of months before I did. Sadly, Catherine became badly ill with puerperal psychosis and really was at times a bit odd and sometimes critical of me. In contrast to myself, she was supported well by her husband, my friend, Jack, who was a social-worker. Over the years of Megan's early childhood, we visited each other a lot, our babies grew very close and their friendship survived into adulthood.

When Megan was about eight months, I had a setback in that my GP, an attractive man called Dr Nielssen, started to take a special interest in me. He would drop in to see me allegedly after he had visited someone else on my stair. He then started to tell me that I had bewitched him. After a few weeks of being besieged by him and being desperately needy and flattered by the interest of a debonair doctor, he persuaded me to go to bed with him. He was a pretty hopeless lover but informed me never-the-less that all my mental problems would now be cured - clearly he had been inspired by some of his Victorian predecessors. He then lent hard on me to be 'good', that is - not to breathe a word about this - he belatedly told me he was married and also could be struck off as a doctor for taking advantage of my ultra-vulnerable state.

Such was his power over me that, when on my next visit, he informed me that I had to change GPs, no choice, in spite of being terribly distraught and feeling cheapened and used by all this, I did not for one moment consider informing on him. This was because I imagined the impact on his wife and children whom I thought did not deserve to pay for his infringement of his medical codes. Moreover I judged myself as complicit rather than abused. I later heard through the grapevine that he had similarly used another woman patient suffering from post-natal depression.

And his abuse of me took its toll, making me further vulnerable to men and even less able to discriminate. I became involved with David, the very mixed-up brother of my sister-in law. Megan was about eighteen months old. However things got very messy. I allowed Lincoln to come to visit us and share Megan's second birthday. He actually crossed paths with David, arriving late one night when David was with me. I could not deal with the situation and took some sleeping tablets, leaving the two men glowering at each other. Next morning David took off. I told him that I was going to try and make things work with Megan's Dad. Lincoln stayed with us for a few weeks and wanted to live with us and to take a role as Megan's father.

However it was winter time and again I did not fully trust his motives. When Christmas was nearing, I approached my mother as to whether Lincoln could come as well to our family Christmas, she said not. So I had to chose to spend a rather straitened time en famille with Megan and Lincoln in my cramped tenement flat or join the family and leave Lincoln on his own. I chose the latter. This was an incredibly selfish choice with no loyalty to Lincoln but I suppose I was still trying to cling to some image of a happy family Christmas for Megan with her grandparents. And I did not want to challenge my mother's controlling prejudices. Looking at this now, I suspect I still desperately wanted her to accept me and my choices unconditionally and could not face the fact that she did not. And it should have been no shock to me that when I got back to Edinburgh for Hogmany with Lincoln, he was gone.

I fell to pieces. Losses have, since Rose's death, always been the trigger for massive crises for me. Catherine came round and, seeing the state I was in, informed my GP and advised my admission into hospital. I actually think now that this was ill-advised but I went in voluntarily for over a week and Megan was looked after by Jack and Catherine.

With what I now regard as typical callous medical indifference to suffering in many "cases" such as mine, I was taken off all the drugs I was on for an 'assessment'. Withdrawing me suddenly from tranquillizers was highly dangerous but fortunately I did not have a fit but was completely strung out and unable to sleep at all.

In my dazed state, I struck up a romance with a very ill young man who visited me for a few weeks after I went back home and tried to pick up the pieces of myself. He was in Carstairs as a schizophrenic patient but was very gentle if a bit stupid but I was in no state to be discerning

Then my brother, Ewan, had the first of a few years of 'psychiatric' problems. In 1976, he was living with his new wife Rhona in an overseas posting in Nigeria but everything went wrong. One of Ewan's best friends out there was killed in a car-crash, Ewan and Rhona took to smoking the extra strong local weed and, according to Rhona, he became out of control and hit her. Eventually he was sectioned and transported back to an English hospital. At this point Rhona abandoned him and never saw him again. I am angry with her to this day but she was still only about twenty-two and no doubt had no understanding of such an illness.

Ewan was later transferred back to Edinburgh. I visited him regularly in the Royal Ed and eventually he came to live with Megan and I to recuperate. He was drooling from the heavy doses of the drug Haloperidol and could barely walk or talk at times. He was terrified of being on his own. He used to have to accompany me everywhere, even on my daily trips up the Royal Mile as I took Megan to school. He would pace up and down at night unable to sleep. I knew only too well what that torture was like. At one point in the middle of the night he asked me in despair what he should do. I asked him if he was contemplating suicide at all, my biggest fear of course - he said he was but would not do it. Then I said all he could do was pray and keep on hanging on.

He did keep hanging on. One day whilst he was with me he met my friend, Mark, with whom I used to practise Tai Chi out in Holyrood Park. Much to my surprise, Ewan took to Tai Chi eagerly. He attended classes at the Salisbury Centre and made huge progress on all fronts, eventually being able to return to employment. He was very disciplined and became qualified to teach. He then decided that he could not progress further with Tai Chi until he was less stiff so he took up yoga which then became his life-long practise to which he devoted a few hours every day, on his own, never in a class. Although he was later diagnosed as a manic depressive and told to take lifelong lithium he refused and Yoga turned him around. A couple of years later when he had a second serious bout of illness, again after heavy use of dope, his psychiatrist told me that his life-expectancy would be lowered so I am extremely grateful that Ewan dedicated himself to yoga as a path of recovery and is still alive today.

At this time I attended a mother-and-toddler group but recognized that I needed to get out of an evening as an adult. I approached the University Settlement which was a project that mobilised student volunteers and through their admirable work, Sheena, a volunteer babysitter, entered our lives like a ray of sunshine. She came regularly once a week like clock-work and Megan came to love her. She let Megan brush her beautiful fair hair for hours. On my nights off, I started to attend the Salisbury centre where I also joined a Tuesday morning dream-work group for mothers of young children run by the prestigious and amazing psycho-analyst, Winifred Rushforth, who was over ninety-five by this time but still imparted much care and wisdom to this band of beleaguered mothers.

When Megan was past one, I requested access to part-time day-care and after a nasty but mercifully short spell with a local child minder, then a dreadful day-care centre, I was lucky enough to get a placement for her in Moray House Montessorri nursery run by a dramatically histrionic Miss Davidson, who lulled the infants to sleep with long poetry recitations. However Miss Davidson was perturbed that in her professional opinion, I took Megan to too many places during the afternoon and was over-stimulating her - she reported that Megan did not drop off to sleep well. She insisted Megan had to attend full-time or not at all, which infuriated me but left me with no choice. I used to take Megan up the Royal Mile on the back of my bike and often she would be chanting "I don't wanna go to nursery school" – awful. Moreover her favourite activity there seemed to have been making chocolate crispies. She did however have one fun friend, the daughter of an interesting couple. He was a Spanish anarchist community artist and she was a language teacher. Their quixotic daughter, Alice, and mine got into trouble with Miss D. for casting spells!!!!

However the nursery place freed me up to do some community work and I became a volunteer at the Tollcross Residents Association. Tollcross at that time was in a dire state and several streets were undergoing reconstruction. They had a small community centre staffed by a dynamic young woman, with whom I worked doing a variety of office jobs and answering queries from the public.

I now was sort of living some sort of functioning life with occasional attempts at romance with passing men who really were not options given my responsibilities to Megan. From then on, her needs acted as a filter to require me to make better choices. Two really important positive things happened at this stage of my life. One was my meeting Libby at the dream-work group. Her little girl, Tessa, was a bit older than Megan but they became fast friends as did Libby and I. She is still to this date my oldest and most loyal friend. At that time she lived out of town in Penicuik with Rajah. They had both recently become sannyasins to Bhagwham Rajneesh and I attended the wild meditations regularly. This enabled me to begin to vent some of the terrific pent-up rage and trauma inside. Libby and Rajah were also incredibly supportive to me and drove us out to their lovely little suburban home regularly for weekends and for seasonal earth festivities. Some of the most lovely memories of my life are of the hours spent in their home and I hope also this was true for Megan. Libby is a very cultured person and so was Rajah and we talked about anything and everything.

As the years went by, Libby's relationship with Rajah became impossible as she became infatuated with a younger sannyasin. I had been his first lover a couple of years before but quickly ended it as he was clearly too much trouble, even for me. Libby's life became increasingly disturbed with time but in those years of our friendship, visits to their home gave me a sense of happy family that I had not got with my own parents.

The other huge change in my life happened through my joining a Woman's Studies Adult Education course at Edinburgh University. The subjects interested me, including women and mental health, women and religion but little did I know that this was not a course like any other that I had attended before. We students had to research, then present, the subjects ourselves. I did 'Women and Madness 'and 'Women and Religion' - the latter led to a real epiphany for me.

For the last year or so I had become mesmerised by religious institutions, having been unwillingly plunged into religious experiences non-stop during my years of insomnia and the emergence of unconscious symbolism. I particularly was fascinated by the Episcopal Church with the colourful runic signs on the cassock of the priest, the dancing motions he made as he processed round the altar. The book "The Paradise Papers" opened a huge door in my mind. It was a real religious experience. Suddenly I realized the monstrous lie – the reversals that Christianity had made, the usurpation of womens' menstrual power and the substitution of empty ritual on the back of earlier pagan festivals. I became in one moment a life-long feminist.

This took visible form in my joining the newly forming Edinburgh Rape Crisis group, the first such group in Scotland. For a couple of years we met in a squalid basement not far from Edinburgh's notorious red-light zone and eventually established a Rape Crisis centre with a help-line staffed by all of us as volunteers. I was not a key member of the group but I did my bit. It was very nerve-wracking taking my first few calls but we tried to work in pairs and used the training offered by the London centre. I even appeared on TV with a small plug announcing our opening.

Equally important was my joining the First of May collective, a radical bookshop in an alley off the Royal Mile.   I helped out on the rota taking Megan with me. We sold a wide range of left-wing and anarchist books and periodicals. As a result of the contacts I made there, I also joined a housing coop composed of many members of the shop.   Some of the Men against Sexism group offered childcare services to unsupported mothers and two men did babysitting for me, for which I was truly grateful.

I was also still trying to deal with my emotional problems, and in the absence of any NHS treatment for trauma, I joined a Gestalt group and a dream drama group, attending the Easter schools at Otterburn of the Sempervivum movement, all facets of the growth movement burgeoning at that time. I did primal rebirthing with an older man called Joe Welowski and at the end of it had an experience of transcendence. The rebirthing consisted of body work and, by turns, we held each other down and we each had to push our way out, all to the deafening sound of taped maternal heartbeats. All in all, a lot was happening for me. With hindsight, I question whether much of this often primal and cathartic therapy really helped 'heal' me and it was of course expensive. Whilst it was wonderfully liberating at first to be given permission to 'cathart', these groups did not offer coaching in non-violent communication or other tools for transacting interpersonal problems. They also evacuated any political content out of participants' distress. But the sorry state of affairs was that there was no other help available for me and I was unwilling to share, even with my close friends, what underlay my often distressed emotional state.

Rajah was a pagan, which resonated with me and he invited me on a trip to Ireland to visit the bizarrely fabulous temple of Isis in Clonegal Castle where I attended his ordination as a priest of the Order. We collected stones from all parts of Britain and Rajah erected a small circle in his garden and began to hold quarterly festivals which I also attended. They were quite sedate affairs and it was a few years till I attended my first full-blooded pagan ceremony.

Then I decided to make a big change in my life. A woman from the First of May bookshop invited me to move into a group-flat with herself and several others from the same network. And I did so quite without, with hindsight, due reflection. I was really exhausted by my isolation as an adult, and struggling alone with a little child and no family back-up. I rented out my flat to another lone parent and moved in with this new group in rented accommodation which we had been assured was secure. My house-mates were mostly academics and all allegedly left-wing. There were two married couples and myself and another single woman, also one other child, a little boy called Laurie.

Overnight my lonely life down in an out-of-the way part of town was transformed, as this flat was in a central part of town in the Meadows and friends found it much easier to visit me. There were good things about this situation but Megan found it really hard to suddenly have to adapt to not having a home where she had me all to herself. She rejected Laurie consistently. He was younger and seemed to be doted on by his Mum but she really did not have much time for him in actuality and he kept coming up to Megan and me wanting to play with us. Megan absolutely did not want this. There were also painful tensions at the meal-table as Laurie's parents required him to eat every morsel on his plate and I did not have the same rule for Megan.

Then I had one or two sexual partners at that time but the main dynamic is that the other single woman house-mate and I became attracted to one of the married men. He was attracted to this other single woman, not myself, but the other married man was attracted to me and blurted this out to his wife. She then was horrible to me backed up the other single woman. These dynamics were never discussed. Then I had a full-on relationship with a member of the SWP, Jim. He thought my flat-mates were stuck-up and in their heads and they, for their part, made it clear that they did not like him. Two of my female flatmates told me that they thought Megan was suffering because of this connection. I thought that they were trying to manipulate me to drop my only ally in the flat but in fact, after a rough time at a rebirthing group that I invited Jim to, I backed off from him- he was fun, sexual but too unreliable.

It was at this point that I started to meditate, having attended lessons given by a lovely man in the Salisbury centre. It had a dramatic effect on me. I knew I could at last come off the sleeping tablets and I did. I had no idea of any safe protocol and just stopped overnight. I then had a nasty fit, which was pretty scary as before I fell to the floor, I had bumped into one of my flat-mates and she suddenly looked uncannily like Rose, my dead sister.

Then seemingly out-of-the blue I was drawn to spend a week at Findhorn community which was about twenty miles from my childhood home. I had heard about it for a while but suddenly and inexplicably the pull became irresistible. And my week there convinced me that I wanted to join. I had an interview with two members of the Personnel Department, stalwart pillars of Findhorn who interviewed me for an hour, an interview which included staring at me in silence for a few minutes. I was told that they could see me there but not at that time. I returned home determined that this would be my next step. And my life began to line up in that way but only after a really desperate period.

The landlord of the Meadows flat gave us all notice to quit. I had nowhere to stay and Megan was due to start Gillespies primary school. I was really stuck. My brother, Ewan, had just bought a little cottage in the

Water of Leith colonies and he had a spare room which he offered us. I leapt at the chance and we moved there, sleeping on a mattress on the floor with all our belongings in boxes around us. But it soon became clear that Ewan was in the midst of another nervous breakdown, was drinking and smoking dope, was manic and impossibly out-of-control. When I challenged him about throwing cigarette butts on the floor near newspapers, risking burning us all to death, he got menacingly angry and I thought he was going to hammer me. But he threw us out and the next day we were on the street, literally.

It was dire. My friend, Shakti, offered me a room in her two-room flat in Abbeyhill. Megan and I resided in one room which had space only for our bed and we had to tiptoe into the main room to get Megan's breakfast so as not to wake Shakti. We ate in bed. As a single person she lived by very different hours. In fact she was not often in the flat spending most nights sleeping with her elderly lover, a Gestalt therapist.

It was hard for me to keep things steady for Megan as she started school and a very emotional time for me as I took her there on her first day. But another change happened then. I had been persuaded by a body-worker to do her training course in postural integration, a form of Rolfing which included emotional release. One of the trainers was called Callum and after a few months, there emerged a strong attraction between us. He was involved with another single parent near where he lived in the north of England. But it became clear after a few weeks that he shared my vision of living in a community. He visited Findhorn and was very impressed. We decided to join up and go together. And in fact, now that I had a man in tow and was no longer a feckless lone parent, the Findhorn doors magically opened.

Until Callum sold his house we decided that Megan and I would move in there with him. But even before this happened, things were not good between us. In fact we had got off to a very bad start. Callum had two-timed me right at the beginning and when I did the same a few weeks later, he turned against me. He also started objecting to the fact that, as I was a lone parent on benefit, when I moved in with him, I would no longer be eligible and he would have to cover my expenses until my flat sold. It became a horrible struggle about money and I should have backed off then. He clearly did not want to share his life fully with myself and Megan. He did however behave very caringly to Megan and she was fond of him. And the fact that we were homeless at this point and I wanted desperately to go to Findhorn as we had planned left me feeling I had to rely on him to get us out of an impasse.

Basically we were not at all compatible. He was stolid Lancashire working-class lad who had got a scholarship to Oxford. He had worked on Concorde then with ICI and next, after the break-up of a second relationship, he dropped out of his professional life, took up body-work and working freelance for North Sea Oil. But though he had decided to embrace the alternative life, he was ultimately quite a conservative and ultimately chronically depressed person. Two of my anti-sexist baby-sitters warned me off moving in with him. They told me they found him oppressive and sexist.

However I went ahead. I was in love with him, I could not go on living in one bedroom and subject Megan to such a makeshift life. And moreover the partnership with Callum was a passport to a new life at Findhorn. However I had to go through a humiliating session with him where Libby sat down with him and explained just how much it costs to support a child. Callum decided to give me an allowance of £30 per week. But not before telling me in anger that he did not want to live with me.

In spite of this, we stuck together and moved shortly to Findhorn to begin a new life as a family and as members of that community. Maybe we went ahead because whilst I was staying with Callum, I accidentally became pregnant. I think Callum so wanted a child that he overlooked our incompatibility and I guess he also loved/hated me.

Strangely at this very time, I was invited to join a very different community, the all-women feminist community at Stanley Road, in Edinburgh. I was clear however that it was Callum and Findhorn for me. Now, I wonder often how my life might have been if I had instead chosen to go to live with a group who had actually asked me to join them, as opposed to going to a community that did not want myself and Megan on our own and with a man who did not ultimately want me as I was.

We lived in Findhorn for two and half years and I learnt such a lot. We became macro-biotic for several years, a horrible change for Megan. This decision was taken on principle by Callum but for health reasons by myself as I had decided that my poor diet was a contributory factor in my depression. I am not to this day decided as to whether these years of detox. really helped or not but certainly reducing my huge addiction to sugar must have prevented some of the later health problems that beset some of my other siblings. But this dietary regime made it harder than ever to fit into 'normal' society.

I worked part-time in the Findhorn publishing company and Callum was at first in Maintenance and then in the pottery. I will not write about the details of our stay there as I have covered that in separate publications. Our little boy, Craig, was born when I was thirty-five and this ushered in a whole new era of our lives. We saw a lot more of my parents who became more closely involved with the children, especially with Megan.

What was clear was that I found living with a partner created huge anxiety in myself and highlighted my complete inability to handle the inevitable conflict of a relationship in anything but in a very distressed way. Callum and I rowed regularly nearly every ten days or so. I often got out-of-control and would scream and throw things. Callum would close down and be cold and cruel. It came to a head when Craig's birth was overdue. Megan was luckily away at that time as any day now I expected to go into hospital. One night in bed Callum and I clashed over his sexual and emotional rejection. I could not stop haranguing him so he got out of our bed and went to try to sleep in Megan's tiny empty bed. I followed him ranting. He reared up suddenly, lifted me up bodily and hurled me back onto our bed. I lay there with my heart thumping and straightaway, my waters broke. I cried out in fear and Callum rushed me into hospital. Just after the birth as I cradled my son in my arms, Callum asked me to look at him as he told me he loved me. I could not answer or look at him. We never spoke about this again.

If I had not been in a community that would have thrown me out as a lone parent, I wonder if I would have had the strength to leave a man who risked not only my life but that of his infant with such an out-of-control act of violence but I doubt I could face up to things with such a backlog of undealt-with issues. And in fact Callum never assaulted me again for five years, which then decided me on ending it all. But at that later juncture, I had fallen in love with someone else and possibly could not have split from Callum without having a new man in my life. But I will come to that sorry tale later.

Summarising these seven years, I can detect some greater stability in my life as I tried to create a home and family for Megan, starting as ourselves as a solo unit, then branching out into group-living then finally doing the whole package, a partner then in a big community. Through all these different phases, however, I carried my distress along.

CHAPTER 6

Times They Are A changing

The next few years were spent getting swept along somewhat belatedly in the tides of change that were part of the 60's generation. I had to adapt to living with a man, surviving in an apolitical New Age community and coping with a screaming colicky son.

Craig burst upon us like a bombshell. Possibly in keeping with his traumatically induced birth, he brought explosive energy into our lives. For the first two weeks, we thought we were truly blessed. Our son had a golden halo of fluffy hair, his head glowed and emanated peace. Whether it was coincidence or not, when I went back to work when he was two weeks old, all hell started to break loose. I was apart from him for three-hour shifts and when he needed to nurse, Callum would wheel him to me in our massive old community-pram. Their progress down from our caravan could be tracked from afar by the terrible squawling racket. In hindsight I should have dropped work but I was never too good at being cooped up with a child for hours on end and the community was not child-friendly. So we persisted in our routine. Callum worked in maintenance and I worked in the accounts section of the Findhorn publishing company.

Megan started at Kinloss Primary School but did not settle there, possibly due more to the unsettling nature of all the change she had had to undergo rather than the rigorous nature of a RAF-dominated school. After a few weeks, I took her out of school and so began four years of 'home schooling' or rather ignoring academic learning altogether. I had tried to introduce reading to Megan when she started primary school and had made a dreadful job of it, expecting her to master learning on a book that was far too complex for a beginner. And in an access of guilt, I took all such stress off her and let her enjoy all the freedom I could. She spent a lot of time around the community when other children were at school. As Craig howled so much and pre-occupied both Callum and myself as parents, she was terribly pushed out. One of my friends thought we were neglecting her as she would go round to her and say 'Mummy'. Horrible to be told that. I tried so hard to give her attention whilst holding a baby that screamed night and day. We instituted "Megan-time", a special slot allocated by both of us adults to give her time one-to-one. Callum did not take to all the demands of this scenario very well and, having been very attentive to Megan before Craig's birth, he could just about manage Craig but had no energy left over for Megan or myself. We could none of us get any peace as the noise of wails went right through the small caravan.

All in all we were in a hard place for the first couple of years. There were some beautiful times. We went on an adventurous sailing holiday with another couple and their two girls and, even though Callum and I and some of the others were seasick, it was something that Callum really enjoyed. I loved sacred dancing and the many beautiful meditations held in the huge community hall. We had a camper-van and went on a tour of Ireland. We had a beautiful naming-ceremony for Craig. And generally tried our very best to make life as good as we could in a difficult setting.

However Callum soon began to hate life at Findhorn and to get restless for a change. He gave up on any hope of the old guard of the community ceding power and he was shocked at the waste of oil and other energy that was necessitated by trying to keep old caravans habitable in the freezing winters. The new attempt at an eco-village back-fired and it became clear to us that the new venture would end up as a luxury eco-village for the well-to-do.

I for my part found the whole model of spirituality really misogynist and Christianized. There were some truly shocking abuses of women and children going on. I became unpopular with the powers-that-be for bringing such matters up. Moreover within the community I landed up very much a lone feminist voice. Some women from the connected garden-school were expelled for questioning power-relations and sexism there. After a while I also agreed with Callum that we should find another community. He was inspired by a group living on the West coast involved in de-schooling their kids. So we packed all our gear into our camper and set off for a new beginning.

This new community of Callum's choice was called Open Sky and was moreover literally open to the sky with a gaping hole in the roof in parts. It was a rented derelict cottage at the end of a track, miles from nowhere. It consisted of one family, a couple and four kids and one single woman with two kids. The single woman was already very disillusioned by the time we got there. I was ensconced with the two children several miles away in a wee cottage on the beautiful

Lunga estate. I knew nobody, the cottage was poorly heated by a demanding and cantankerous Aga, we arrived in mid-winter and it was a real struggle for me with two little children and no outside contact, not even a phone.

The following chilling misadventure illustrates the rigours of our new life. One day, overcome with isolation, I even set off with the kids through the snow to trek the few miles along the coast to Open Sky and we got caught in a blizzard. We landed up completely lost and exhausted, I was having to carry a heavy toddler and it was only by sheer luck that I managed to get us back. For a couple of hours, I thought we would not make it and would die together in the snow.

So we lasted there a few months and then decided to retreat back to the north-east and camp in an ancient caravan on the croft of some friends near Keith. They had also de-schooled their two children but were following a Steiner approach. The caravan had no running water and was very basic, mouldy and damp. Again it was a real struggle. We had to bath Craig in a small blue bucket. Also the woman of the house was not really at all friendly and Megan, who was lonely for company, was not always welcome to play with her kids, even when they wanted her to.

Callum's Dad came to visit us. A quiet aloof man, he took stock of the situation swiftly. His last words to his son were "Take care of them, Callum." Callum was however as blinded by idealism as I was – either that or we knew we could not be happy en famille. We both thought community-life was the answer and decided to embark on a tour of the ones we had selected from the directory of alternative communities as those most suited to our de-schooled and dietary approach.

This proved quite an adventure but did not lead to a community home for us. The best of the bunch was called Holme Place and was in Devon and later moved to Wales- they were into de-schooling and family beds and I got the idea they were also a set of swinging couples, none of whom appealed to me. We had some nasty shocks in Ireland where, on my wishes, we visited briefly at An Dreochad Beo, allegedly a matriarchal community for women and children, possibly men as well. It was rigidly hierarchical and we found out later that there was S&M going on. As it happened Sister Boss took to us as much as we took to her and we beat a hasty retreat.

Our next port of call was in their neighbouring community on Innisfree island, Atlantis, with Becky and Snowy James and their terrified entourage. We stayed there three days and, though we had known it was a primal scream community, this was not structured but was basically a free-for-all. I apparently did well in their hierarchy given my venting background. The James sisters, however, were highly insulting about Callum being 'pussy-whipped' because he took care of our son half-time and they blamed him for Craig's screaming. We had a show-down with them or, I should say, eventually I mutinied, refusing to spend a morning washing men's socks by hand. Callum was too scared to speak but I said we wanted to leave. However they told us that we would have to find our own way off the island – swimming? Eventually one of the saner men rowed us off. Phew!

After that anything for a quiet life as far as I was concerned. On our trip to Lauriston Hall community in Dumfries and Galloway, we worked out that this would not suit us but we found out about a local school which was a free-school, loosely following the A. S. Neill model. This inspired us and we decided to buy a wee run-down cottage near the school in a village.

So just before Christmas of 1987 we moved there for our new life, home-building. I ended up living there for over twenty years or so but it became clear after a couple of years that Callum had seen this home only as a temporary expedient, given that we had been at our wits-end, basically homeless, touring in a camper, looking for a Nirvana to replace our tarnished Findhorn. It also became painfully clearer to me that Callum was never going to face the fact that children needed a regular life and regular money coming in.

From then on my life with him became a continual financial struggle trying to make ends meet and dealing with the endless ordeal of signing on the dole. Callum claimed I could be the one to go out to work but basically I still had a dependent two-year old son and a nine-year old daughter who had become a day-pupil at Kilquhanity. Being basically a private school, the children has twenty-six weeks holiday a year and child-care was an issue in relation to a job. For me as well there were no jobs in the village and it took me a year to pass the driving test belatedly at age thirty nine. But the local town had no jobs either that fitted in with the needs of the kids. It became a hard way of life with my nagging Callum to do his bit, him working part-time at Kilquhanity for £30 a week and us supplementing   this   with   working-tax-credit   or whatever deal the government of the day was operating.

Thus I was still stuck very much outside the camaraderie of a work-team and in the role of mother, with its isolation and drudgery very depressing for someone already depressed. Callum also was probably isolated and depressed but saw the answer as joining another community. This became more of an issue as Megan settled in school, I made feminist friends, at first through a playgroup, then through a local group of mainly lesbian women who had settled a few miles away in an old farmhouse. They were pretty radical in such a conservative area and although not a lesbian and thus fully one of them on their terms, I shared more in common with them than with the locals and pretty soon my social life was tied up with their circle.

Meanwhile I got swept away in another development of feminism in the confrontation over Cruise missiles on Greenham common. This initiated myself and a swathe of others in a whole new way which brought together radical politics and spirituality. I was present at that amazing day, in December 1983, the Embrace the Base happening – fifty thousand women linking hands around the perimeter fence and camping there for ten days. A strong group of Galloway witches formed and there began a few years of earth rituals, women chanting, dancing and improvising ceremonies, reclaiming a bodily and earth-based spirituality, a do-it–yourself approach which was also publicly visible in the rise of Starhawk* in the USA and the American periodical for women, Woman Spirit Rising. (*Starhawk – radical feminist activist who integrated direct action with ritual)

I became a friend of the Goddess champion, Sylvie, at a pagan gathering where I also had a brief intense and influential fling with a transvestite feminist man, Robyn. Sylvie was something of a bigwig in a movement that was ideologically opposed to leaders. She painted prodigiously and also wrote influentially, mainly on Goddess feminism. Eventually she co-published an alternative best-seller on the subject. We were all drawn together by our politics and paganism.

I had the amazing experience of taking part in a huge week-long march of women across the Avebury plain, which included a protest-march for a day across Ministry of Defence land, which was used as a firing range, in a band of around two hundred, including Sylvie and Starhawk (with whom I and some others of the Galloway group were arrested - we shared a police-van and later a campfire for a few hours.) We did however manage to break through the fence into Stonehenge for a wild women's celebration at the stones, probably the first women-only gathering there for centuries, but paradoxically fenced in by a whole group of policemen. It was a full moon lunar eclipse and the middle of the night. I often wonder what the police made of the drumming wild chanting. As we were by this stage all rather grubby and dishevelled from camping out for a few days, they probably wrote us off as mad.

All this was tremendously exciting for me but of course did not include Callum. He held the fort for me on my trips away. He could and did however attend Green gatherings in England with the children and we looked forward to them but they made little impact on his general low mood. We were jointly part of a pagan group called PAN (Pagans Against Nuclear Energy) and spent a week camping with the group in Sherwood Forest, culminating in a huge ceremony. With a small dose of mushrooms this was a potent occasion for me as it was the first time I had been in a mixed-sex pagan circle. Bel, a handsome muscled young stud, danced round the circle drumming, offering us the blood and body of the mother in sacramental wine and bread. I was in an exalted realm.

But back to the prosaic everyday reality of home. Callum made no real effort to integrate anywhere in the region and became very bitter towards life and me. Never a demonstrative man, he became positively withholding towards myself and Megan and there were regular furious rows, from which I tried to shelter the kids. However they inevitably witnessed some of them in which I did my utmost to control myself but it must have been horrible and scary for them. I have huge guilt over the scenarios I exposed them to as children but I tried my utmost to do the best I could to shield my children from our traumatised and traumatizing rows.

We carried on in this way for five more years together, Megan settling in Kilquhanity. Craig, when he was old enough, started at a local village school. Because of bullying, which the Head utterly failed to address, we eventually took Craig out of there and he also settled happily in Kilqhanity.

There was a period that was worse than usual about two years after we had settled in Galloway when I had had enough and Callum decided to leave and stay with a self-styled anti-sexist man in a cottage a few miles away. At first it seemed to improve matters. I got a few days break from childcare and the rows were not so intense. But a few weeks into this phase, I was just getting ready to go to Greenham when I got a phone call to say that he was alright but Craig was in hospital. He had been seriously bitten by the dog in the cottage next to Callum's new home. The dog had never bitten anyone before but had apparently found the body of a dead lamb. Nobody could tell how the attack happened but I suspect Craig ambled along to the dog who maybe had a bit of the carcass. Anyway I rushed into Dumfries. My little boy had been bitten deeply in the top of his forehead and the back of his neck and right through his hand. He was just about to get stitched up when I got there.

Callum and I were into co-counselling at this point and one of its tenets was that people should not have anaesthetics but cry their way through the pain in order that the pain does not get locked into cellular memory. Well, we insisted on that for Craig. We were not allowed into the operating-theatre but I ignored the doctor and barged in as Craig was crying for me. I held Craig's unbitten hand whilst he had ten minutes or so of stitching. The doctors were shocked and insisted in a tight-lipped fashion that Craig was to be given antibiotics.

Craig should officially have gone back to Callum that night and I was all set to head off south. I kept him with me over the night however and then went off as arranged but now I wonder how I could have been so selfish as to leave a three year-old after such an ordeal. I did however trust Callum completely to take real good care of him.

However living on my own with two children in the country, things got really awful for me as I was left with a whole group of new problems. I also got carried away in a tide of anger towards Callum's new landlord friend, Nick. His ex-wife was furious that he had decamped with a whole library of her feminist books and spent many hours venting her righteous rage towards the whole scene at his house. This included Nick having a continuous string of women under the guise of 'unconditional loving' and I, for my part, feared this would contaminate both Callum and Craig. So one afternoon, I 'liberated' all the feminist books to form a library for local women.

I thought his rageful ex-wife would be delighted but what happened next shows just how thin this man's anti-sexism was and I was undermined in that his ex did a volte-face and shunned me. She could not believe what I claimed Nick next did. However at first I had the backing of my local feminist friends until Nick reported me to the RSPCC as a risk to my children under various counts, including that I was a witch and forced my son to wear girls' clothes.

The RSPCC official visited us and established from me that I knew I had an enemy. He told me that he had made investigations round the village but had found no grounds for concern. And he named the call as malicious and made by Nick. I was utterly devastated. Moreover my feminist allies, mostly lesbians, suddenly fell away in their support for me. As lesbian mothers they feared this anti-sexist stalwart might act against them next. I was left on my own with this. Moreover, Nick chucked Callum out of his house, as his presence there had given me access. So Callum was back at home with us. I made Nick's malicious call public in anti-sexist circles and, to my horror and anger, met with a wall of blind disbelief - all that is apart from the solidarity of Robyn and a friend of his called Des, who was at that time partner to Sylvie - later Des became key to my life.

Des and Robyn formed a support-group for me and took on the public face of unmasking Nick. However inspite of Des's dogged campaign on my behalf, all that happened was that my name was further blackened. After a year of harrowing letters from 'anti-sexist' men I gave up. Callum and I split up again after a few months and he got a cottage by himself a few miles away but had to return when the Dept. of Social Security cut him off.

Another of my involvements was as part of the Snowball campaign. This was an explicit attempt to gain legal ground by taking a token action against nuclear bases, like trying to cut the wire of a Ministry of Defence fence, getting arrested and then arguing the legal case in court. This culminated in several of our Galloway group coming to trial in a court case in Cumbria re Windscale and being given a chance to read out our defence in court. My friend gave a fiery but factual tirade. I gave an emotional weepy one. We got off with a fine in the end.

Another time we went off to an action against Trident at Faslane and drove back in a snow-storm. We got stuck overnight in a snow-drift in Ayrshire, five women activists and my little Megan. There was panic in the ranks at one point, with one woman losing control of her bowels, luckily in a plastic bag, much to the disgust of our driver who was stolidly reading

Emma Goldman's "Life of a Revolutionary." The panic was triggered when our car, already covered half-way up the doors, was struck by a snow-plough. I hoped the driver would notice but he drove on. I tried to get out of the car to chase after him and let him know of our plight. But a furious snow-filled wind choked me and the others yelled at me to get back in the car. We were left skewed half across the road unable to get out and a sitting target for any other vehicle.

Luckily the road was closed after that and we stayed there as the snow steadily rose until it covered the roof. The other women went to sleep but I stayed awake to keep digging an air-passage for us out of the window. I remember at the height of the drama having panic rising in my stomach and thought I was going to go to pieces but I had Megan with me and her needs focussed me. When one overwrought passenger started sobbing and holding onto me asking "Are we all going to die?" I said 'No.' I told myself inwardly that if we did die, at least I would show dignity and put all my energy into making what might be the last few hours of Megan's young life untroubled. It was a very long and hungry cold night but we were found about five in the morning, wakened by the loud singing of some drunken male revellers walking along the top of the drift on their way home. At that point, a rift broke out in the car as one woman did not want us to yell for help in case we got raped!! But she got shouted down. Soon we were ensconced in a miner's cafe with rolls and tea.

It was at a pagan gathering around 1985 that I became further involved with Robyn in a very compulsively hypnotic relationship where I was intrigued by his sexual ambiguity, cross-dressing and intensity. I then visited him in London where he lived at that time. I took Megan with me to see her Dad and to visit some of the London sights. Robyn then came up to our cottage and stayed for a few days. Such was the estrangement by this time between myself and Callum that I saw fit to ask him how he would feel if I slept with Robyn under the same roof. He said "Go right ahead" so I did. My relationship with Robyn, however, did not last long. I found him too obsessed with his gender-identity, too volatile and unable to connect with my needs to parent my children, not him.

However he moved to Wales a short while after. This was to live with Des who had been left by Sylvie after their family was hit by double-tragedy. Over the couple of years that I knew her, Sylvie had poured out to me her troubles with Des, particularly about his role as stepfather to her teenage son, Eric. However at this point, Eric got killed in a road accident in France, then Sylvie's second son developed lymphatic cancer and took over a year to die. Sylvie left Des and went to live in Bristol to be near her sick son.

I visited Sylvie in Bristol. She was understandably in a dreadful state and full of rage against Des, who had almost acquired diabolical dimensions now that Eric was dead. She said that a few months before the tragedy, Des had yelled at Eric that he should have been aborted. Sylvie said that it was due to his anxiety at coming home to Des that Eric did not look properly at the traffic before he rushed under a car. She also blamed separatists for his death, in that Eric had been upset over their questioning that such a maturing lad as he was should be in the women's camp in France.

I went to Bristol on my way to visit Robyn who had in fact moved into a dilapidated cottage in Wales with Des. This was the second time I had seen Des, the first was a brief encounter at a green-gathering when I had banged into him as he was circling the camp trying to round up men for the crèche. I spotted him across a field and felt a visceral jolt. Now I was to stay in the home of this charismatic man who had put so much effort into supporting me through the Nick struggle – he was also the man about whom I had heard so much anguish and who was to bring a double dose of it into my life as well.

It was predictable that I fell for him, hook-line-and sinker. I rejected Robyn's distressed advances. It became clear to the three of us what was developing but I did nothing to betray Sylvie or Robyn. I did however give a lot of time to listening to Des as he lay in bed weeping loudly of a morning over the loss of Eric.

I then went home and tried to put Des out of my mind but I had pretty intense fantasies about him. Our paths were not to cross for a couple of years. My uneven life in Galloway continued. I got involved in shamanic work with some of the Galloway gals and a travelling shaman. These times were very powerful, including sweat-lodges. The kids progressed.

Then Callum's dad died. He had seen him hardly at all over his adult life and did not seem upset. He did not even set off on his motor-bike early enough to reach the funeral in time. But I noticed that, after this loss, his mood deteriorated. He did teach me to drive however and by this time in 1985, I was able to get about without him.

Then he fell off his motor-bike one night and fractured his collar-bone. All in all he was in a bad way. He talked constantly of wanting to move to a community as the answer to his low feelings. The kids were really settled and so was I, apart from our conflicts, the fact that we had non-stop financial struggle and I felt continually rejected by him. In fact I was repeatedly made to feel undesirable by his cold contempt of my emotionally-driven sexual overtures. I judged that I had failed to make him happy.

The community he settled on as his new Mecca was called Cynlas. It was based in mid-Wales and was in fact the core-group from Holmes Place, who had moved to the country and taken up physical immortalism. Callum went to visit and decided he wanted to move there and for us to come along. I was really dead-set against such a move and moreover my parents in the north were getting older. He grew more restless, angry and rejecting by the day.

I busied myself with the children and my women friends, my shamanic exploits including one bizarre trip away to the shores of Loch Ness to take part in a jamboree called the Harmonic Convergence with my women's group on the land held by the male self-styled guru, Neil Oram. Our camp was run by the Dianic witch, Jean Freer, with a lovely wee sweat-lodge, mask-making and fun, but also a power–clash with Neil Oram. At one point he sent an ultimatum for all feminists to leave his land. Needless to say, we stayed put. I remember lots of laughs including hysteria when Jean's solemn declaration of the charge of the Goddess - "Listen to the words of the Great mother" were met with a resounding fart by Libra.

Then early in 1988 I attended a shamanic camp near New Galloway. This proved powerfully triggering for me as I had a crush on the leader as was sometimes my unfortunate habit with male gurus. I thought he had shacked up for the night with my friend but he had not. I got home around 2 p.m and shortly after, the phone went. I got the news that my father had died. I was in an altered state after the workshop and we all set off up to Speyside to be with my mother. Megan did not however want to come so I left her with a friend.

My father had been in decline for several years with dreadful depression and horrible aggressive moods. He was increasingly plagued with poor physical heath, overweight from the drugs and over-eating and drinking. He was in hospital for angina at the end of 1987. At one point his doctor asked me to get his sleeping tablets off him – the poor young man was exhausted and could not cope any longer with my father's bad temper. I told Dad what I was doing and why. And he yelled at me "Don't do that, you bitch", almost his parting words to me. I was humiliated and ashamed of him as there was a young man unfortunate enough to be parked in a bed next to him and he was seriously ill with heart-failure.

When Dad came home, I remember him once asking me if I was happy. I wanted to say "How could I be after the damage you inflicted on our lives?" But I felt too sorry for him so I said "Well you know me. I'm up and down." He sighed and said I was just like him and that he thought I was too clever for men.

Just before this I had had an out-of-body experience where my father's 'fetch' came to me, running from his car towards me. I yelled "Don't run, Dad, you will have a heart attack" so it was no surprise to me when I heard the news of his sudden death. My first feeling in walking into the dining-room where his body was laid out was of sweet revengeful rage and then the thought "Thank God, now you can't hurt us any more." My mother was terribly upset about his loss, told me how lovely Dad had been at the start. I supported her as best I could. Margaret did not come home for the funeral - she was abroad.

Then I heard that Des had moved to Edinburgh with Robyn as he wanted to be near his eighteen year old daughter, Astrid, who had come to study there. He asked me if I wanted to come to a weekend CND conference and I went accompanied by my friend, Melanie. In the evening there was a dance. About the end I was dancing with Des and Mel - she knew I was crazy about Des and she tactfully slipped away. My heart stopped still. Des had reached out and grabbed my hand. I almost died with happiness. A new chapter in my life was about to start.

I think Callum may have picked up on my happiness. Anyway three weeks after the death of my father, he said he wanted to leave shortly to live in the community in N. Wales that I really could not resonate with because of its New Age orientation. I said "Oh, please, no. My father has just died." He snarled "Just how long are you going to need?" and started to walk out of the room. I threw myself in front of the door. I was on the floor and he kicked me furiously on the legs several times. I was badly bruised.

So when he told me a few weeks later, after weeks of agonizing, that his commitment was to me and the kids and he was staying with us, I told him it was too late. My future would be with Des. It was time for Callum to leave.

CHAPTER 7

A Roller-Coaster Ride with an Anti-Sexist Man

And leave is what Callum did in late summer 1988. He spent a few months readying himself with some trips down to Wales to prepare. On those weekends and others Des came down. On the actual day of Callum's departure, I managed myself well, waving him off on the train calmly enough, with a few sad tears, but able to fondly wish him well. His little seven-year old son was with me waving away. I do not think things really hit Craig for three years or so. At that point, once after I had collected him from a trip down to Callum's, he burst into tears and told me he missed him, his father.

Des was due to move in on the 1st Feb 1989 and I was to have a few weeks on my own with the children. But when Callum came up to visit Craig at Guy Fawkes night, staying with friends nearby, as we walked down the local High Street in a bonfire night procession, I knew something had changed and I knew what. Her name was Edna. Paradoxically I went to pieces. I fell apart in front of Craig and was hysterical.

The next few weeks were hell. That weekend I rampaged up to the house where Callum was staying with friends, haranguing him in front of them – Callum's man-friend said that he could not understand why I was so upset when I had a new partner. He did not realize that the heart is not logical. And in reality of course I had not long lost my Dad and could not cope with the loss of Callum on top of that. I don't now know if I ever did get over him. He was cold and seemingly indifferent to myself and Megan a lot of the time, he assaulted me badly twice but I did sense at some level that he loved me. And the news of his new affiliation rocked my world. It also rocked Des's – he was utterly destabilized to see me in pieces over Callum.

In such a desperate pitch was I that I even badgered Megan to beg Callum to cool it off with Edna until I was more settled. She tried with all her might, also pleading with him that Craig was only seven. But Callum stood firm. I shudder with shame to think I put my poor daughter, who was also, I am sure, suffering terribly, through this spectacle and ordeal.

Moreover I got locked in a struggle with Callum about maintenance, which was all the more bitter as it was fuelled also by the rage of loss. It took weeks of angry letters and phone calls to sort out. Moreover I even banned Callum from seeing Craig till he sorted this out. Edna wrote to me trying to say how I should be glad he wanted to see his son. Her son's father wanted nothing to do with him. I went beserk that she did not show solidarity with me and in the letters I subsequently sent to Callum at his new community-home, I scrawled on the envelope for all to see things like "This man beat me up" and "Scabby Slit" over her lack of solidarity with me.

Happily one of the men of Cynlas, Mark, stepped in between us and asked me what would make it work for me. I said £30 a week maintenance, which Callum was refusing to pay. Callum's position was that Des should pay me this sum as rent, and to cover the fact that he, Callum, had signed over the house to me until Craig was 18. This was correct but Des refused to pay any rent to me. So I was caught between two rigid and patriarchal men. I also believed Callum only signed over the house to me because, if he had not, he would have been forced to sell it if he applied for welfare benefits and he did not want Craig turfed out of his home. Anyway Mark then guaranteed that I would get the £30 sum via the community account.

I went back to my Speyside home at Christmas very broken and often weeping. On the train-journey up our dog had diarrhoea all over a young man's trousers. He took it wonderfully well but that messy episode symbolises the mess I felt I was in and was creating. For the first time in my life on that trip, my mother held me and told me she loved me. I thought bitterly "It is too late to tell me this now" for I could feel nothing. But I did rally, especially as soon Des would be beside me and I could stabilise from the trauma of loss.

Then began over 10 years of an intense relationship which left me even more scarred. My first few months with Des, visiting each other, had been marred by spectacular ups-and-downs, mainly to do with his moods and my over-reactions to them. He had previously been a regular dope-user but I insisted he drop that completely before he moved in with us. Given all the warnings I had about him, I had negotiated a live-in contract with him which also included provisions for non-violent communication with the children. But when he was low he found fault with my kids whose errors he attributed to my 'weak' (i.e. non-authoritarian) mothering. But then he would apologize with profuse tears and win his way back into my affections. Had he come clean before he moved in, he would never have been allowed to darken my door. But he saved the full force of his venom until he was established in my home, my life and my affections.

The pattern that emerged was that he would pick on me for any naughtiness or untidiness of the children. He told me I was an inadequate mother. Moreover he resented any money spent on the children, even though it came from child-benefit and maintenance. The first time it happened was over the fact that Megan sometimes forgot to clean the bath. He cast this as 'wilful disobedience.' On one heated occasion he insisted I should drag her down by the hair, if needed, to make her do it. He cited this as the tactic of his friend, Hannah, who lived in Teepee Valley. Immediately the words were out of his mouth, I went hysterical. I was shouting at him. I was standing in his way at a door. He seized me by the hair, dragged me across the room and he kicked me hard several times on the leg. He then stormed out. I lay there stunned. This horrific pre-cursor of things to come occurred when the children were not at home.

What I think happened at this stage is that it sent me into a PTSD denial. I seemed to put this assault into one bit of my head and got up to go after him to get him to back down. Of course he would not do so for a couple of hours after such a raging row. I insisted that if he did not at once enter counselling he was to leave. He agreed to do that. But it seemed not to have any effect on his conduct and I went into the Stockholm Syndrome. I could not live without his intermittent lavish love and affection. Even on one occasion when my friend, Melanie, walked in and found me lying on the floor crying and I told her what had happened, reality did not break through. Melanie confronted Des. He admitted it and said it would not happen again. But it did. And I slowly began to go under, at the same time living a lie as a feminist.

I also justified the situation by saying to myself that the kids did not see these assaults - I tried to make sure the fights were restricted to times the kids were out. That was of course to ignore the damage the violence was doing to me and thus on my capacity to act as a stable mother. Moreover they did witness several very scary screaming matches, during many of which I was hysterical.

This was the backdrop but on the surface, life with him was good. We loved each other the rest of the time. He did childcare whilst I did a course on dream-work once a week in Edinburgh. He did not want to work in any earning-capacity as he saw his political anti-nuclear work as his contribution to society and at that time we could sign on without too much hassle. We did this for two years - however the money was tight.

The first few years were marked also by big family events which added to the strains on our relationship. First there was my grandmother's 100th birthday which should have been a wonderful weekend. Sadly it was also spoiled by an awful accident whilst we were all getting ready for the celebration in the Craigellachie Hotel. My brother, Ewan, reversed the car and injured his toddler daughter, Alice, who had followed him out of the front door under his wheels. The injury looked dreadful. The back of her head was all caved in.

I focussed much of my energy on trying to keep my mother coping. When she saw her injured granddaughter she started to have what looked to me like a heart-attack. I seated her and told her calmly that Alice would be alright though I had doubts. I kept on soothing her but was aghast when she blasted out violently "I knew they would kill her somehow."

Meanwhile the guilty pair set off fast to Aberdeen hospital with their bleeding daughter held by Elizabeth. The rest of us proceeded to the hotel where all of the many guests were waiting.

In order not to spoil Grandma's big day, my Mum, now back in hostess mode, insisted we had to carry on with the party though we did not know if Alice would live or die. Grandma was on no account to be told. But amidst all the festivities she did of course notice that Ewan was not there and kept asking for him. We just fobbed her off somehow. Alice made it through the day. The next day we all breathed in relief. She was going to make it, though she would have to stay in hospital for a few days. There was a lovely party in Craigellachie village school in Grandma's honour, attended not only by all the little kids but also by key adults in the village who knew Grandma. It was lovely. The highlight of it for Grandma was when Ewan managed to leave the hospital and come to the school. How Grandma's face lit up. For me however the occasion symbolised a key aspect of our family-life in that that even a family celebration went horribly wrong.

Now I need to move the spotlight onto Megan who was entering adolescence when Des arrived in our midst. She moreover had come with me to London to see her Dad and at that point I had a knowing that he was not going to live much longer, even though he assured me that he was using clean needles and the right doses. I felt that I had better prepare Megan for such an eventuality by breaking to her the news that her Dad had an addiction problem. This was not long after the death of her Granddad, of whom she had seen the better parts. She was quite upset by his loss.

Over the next couple of years my accommodating sweet–natured daughter transformed into a sulky and often rebellious teen. She was still attending Kilquhanity, which I later found out involved a lot of premature sexual pressure. Whatever the factors were, I had a deep hunch that Megan was very troubled. I tried to keep communication going in loving style but she shut down on me. For the next couple of years, whilst she was still at home, I was dogged by deep anxiety about what was wrong and this was fuelled by the fact that Rose had developed troubles in adolescence, ending tragically.

I insisted that Megan attend sessions with Sydney, a clinical psychologist whom I was seeing. This followed on my discovering that she was shinning down the roof out of her bed-room window and hitching in to Dumfries with a friend for goodness knows what. I also had been told by a friend at Lauriston Hall that a thirteen year old Megan was seen being 'humped' at a party there by a much older local lad. Of course she hotly denied this. And she somehow convinced Sydney that all was o.k. We at least managed to reach agreements about her going out at night which ensured her safety.

However, as family events piled on, the stress on her multiplied. Fast on the heels of each other came death after death. I had taken her to see her Dad in early 1990 and the visit had been o.k. for a few days. Then Lincoln started drinking. Megan got scared and asked me to take her away. We left fast. That was the last she saw of her Dad.   By this time Megan had left Kilquhanity and tried a few weeks at a local High School. However it soon came out that she had been playing truant. She told me she had been in the toilets in the town all day. What a plight! She decided next to do a Youth Training course in horsemanship at a College in Edinburgh. So at sixteen she left home. I deposited her in the residence and drove off in tears at this watershed. And the fact that I had nobody with whom to share my grief with made it all the more searing. Certainly Des was not at all empathetic. His problems got in the way of bonding with Megan.

She went from the college to work at a stables in Edinburgh. And six months later I had the dreadful task of going there with Des and her friend Astrid to break the news of her Dad's death. It was one of the worst moments of my life to see her face go into a mask of dread. She said that, on seeing us, she thought Craig had died. She also quickly expressed sadness for Lincoln's two other children who had lived with him. Lovely Astrid added "Poor you too, Megan."

She and I attended the funeral in London. She had a panic attack on the underground but managed to make it. But she never openly expressed the full extent of her loss and indeed was quite scathing about any tears I shed, accusing me of melodrama or always trying to steal the limelight. I in fact was devastated by Lincoln's death but more was to come. We had no sooner got back from the funeral than one of my oldest man friends was stabbed to death at Nottinghill

Carnival. Another funeral for me. I returned home and tried to act as mother to Craig whilst in a turmoil of worry over Megan.

Then five months later, my grandmother died, which probably did not impact on Megan too much but, straight after, my Mum died in early January. I think Megan was very upset by this. My Mum had been a kindly figure to her and showed her special love but there was little outward show of grief from Megan and in fact she could not face attending the funeral. Now within two years she had lost four special figures in her life. I was really on high alert.

Moreover I was toiling with all the rows and violence from Des. We had developed a dreadful precarious existence, where he would periodically leave me, I would fall apart, frantically seek then eventually find him. Then we would try again and redouble our visits to therapists. The latter in fact all proved hopeless in dealing with the dynamics of domestic violence, which did not really seem to enter, let alone centre, in their concerns.

Megan then at one point decided to come home for a while. She was dreadfully low. Her friends had all left the area, she had nothing to focus on and did not know what she wanted to do next. Eventually she decided on more riding-training. I cannot remember which came first. I think it was a 3 months course at Glen Eagles equestrian centre followed by a year-long course at the de Montfort University in the English Midlands.

But all the while I knew that she was in desperate difficulties. She was also seriously in debt to me. She was meant to ring me regularly but often did not. Then matters came to a head. She rang me in a state of distress, blurted out that she had bulimia then slammed down the phone. I was in total panic. But it did explain the money troubles and all the other problems. Shortly after, she came back home in her car driven by her boyfriend of the time who was clearly trouble. He moreover had sold her the car which was a danger to drive. She did end it with him or perhaps he did with her, I don't know.

I cannot remember the exact details but she wanted to move to Edinburgh as soon as she could. She got a job in childcare. I insisted she go for therapy. The NHS had no treatment available. I paid for her to see a private therapist. She then had a boy-friend in Edinburgh who was in fact a lad from Galloway whom I liked. But after eighteen months or so that ended and badly. Megan hated him from then on. I am not sure what the issues were but one of them was the fact that he used pornography. She found a job as a live-in nanny. And shortly after she met Daniel. She moved in with him pretty soon and married him after a year or so, terribly young and in a wedding in New York which did not sound very happy. She was in tears the day before as she still had not got a dress she liked. My poor beloved Megan. How I wish I could have given you a better start, a better family-life, the lot.

But I have skipped over what was happening to the rest of us left at home. We ploughed on. I managed to write a political satire about the New Age scene funded by a six months job-creation scheme, in which I was self-employed as a writer.

Craig matured and left Kilquhanity by his own choice at twelve to attend the local High School. This made a big difference to his confidence as he began to be one of the village-boys.   He was however always insecure about his position there as he was a newcomer in their scene. He hung out with his friends in the village, always the last to go home. He had entered the state-system dreadfully behind, with reading and maths score-levels of a seven- year old. He soon caught up however, though after the first few months, he did not apply himself much to his studies.   I suspect his teenage year were really anxious ones, grappling with the undercurrents - and sadly occasionally with open warfare - between myself and his stepfather.

The lives of my sisters and brother were also showing the huge scars that untreated childhood trauma leaves on adult life. Ewan's second marriage was to a very damaged Bangladeshi woman, Yasmin, who had been his house-servant when he worked for a few years in Vietnam. Aged twelve, she had run away from her village home, where she had been tied outside like a dog. She had to escape to avoid a forced marriage to an old man. She reached Hanoi where she worked as a house-servant eventually landing up pregnant to one of her employers, my brother, Ewan.

Ewan was advised by other ex-pats to pay Yasmin off but this attempt failed - Yasmin ran up to the roof of the house and threatened to throw herself off. Ewan understandably, given his background, caved in to this threat of suicide. This was the start of an eventual tormented marriage which had the consolation of producing three lovely girls. The family eventually moved back to Britain and I began to have regular contact with their situation. However this was excrutiatingly painful for me as Ewan would often pour out endless anguish to me- Yasmin could not control her temper and was abusing the two older girls. Ewan said he had often walked down the street with a toddler whose face was badly scratched. I was horrified and urged him to get outside support but he never did. I then agonised for a couple of years as to whether I should contact the relevant authorities.

Eventually I witnessed Yasmin scratching Alice viciously on the face. I intervened immediately, letting Yasmin know that such behaviour to a child was not legal in Britain. She defiantly stated she did not care. I had heard and seen enough and contacted the local Social Work Department. They investigated but stated they found no cause for concern. Presumably Ewan covered up what was happening. For years my intervention in this situation blighted my relationship with Ewan who was very bitter to me about it.

Moreover my younger sister had troubles of her own, with her marriage to an alcohol-dependant husband coming to a difficult end. After the death of our father she started to talk to myself and Margaret about memories she had of possibly being abused sexually as a very young child. She recounted a memory which was particularly troubling her and although I could not myself remember any specific incident, I did have a nasty feeling about all this, especially a very fragmented memory of my own. Elizabeth also told me how our father in his later years often seemed sexually suggestive, trying to kiss her on the lips, and even telling her that in some societies incest was acceptable.

In later years Margaret's life also fell apart and indeed the lives of all of us offspring of my parents illustrate only too graphically what happens when childhood trauma is not addressed. I and each of my siblings needed much medical interventions during all of our adult lives, expensive and all of it ineffective as not addressing our core issues. But back to my life in those years in Galloway.

My functioning went downhill rapidly under all this adversity. Having been running groups in the local community centre for women as part of the self-help movement, I now barely managed to limp along, with most of my activity home-centred. After two years of zero financial input I insisted that Des start to pull his weight on the money-front. He started to work as a free-lance gardener and he used the car. Thus I was usually marooned at home most days. He worked for nine months of the year for four days a week and put money into the house to cover his keep. He however insisted he was being exploited, though he paid zero for accommodation and only put anything into the house when his mother died - then he bought £1,500 worth of household goods. I was never allowed to forget that.

Most of the rest of his energy was put into his anti-nuclear work which was channelled through a group of which he was a key member, the World Court project, which aimed to get a World Court ruling on the legality or otherwise of nuclear weaponry. This campaign was not in fact supported by the CND or the wider peace movement - they saw it as a waste of energy with a predictable outcome. However for Des it was a holy crusade. He travelled extensively and frequently to meetings but in fact the centre of group operations was based in my dilapidated cottage which now received letters addressed to the Institute for Law and Peace, a travesty given what was happening under its roof. His family I found appalling snobs who rarely deigned to visit, his daughter was very painfully aloof and came only to criticise him, though I thought her complaints were highly justified. He acted very divisively about his family, excluding me from visits and the like. The whole focus of the household for me became how to manage emotionally and financially with a violent partner who was obsessed with his political standing.

However what was locking me in most of all were the huge amounts of joie de vivre and affection Des evidenced in his up-moods. We regularly had wonderful walks in the weekends, he played football and romped with Craig and his friends, we went sledging, we used to laugh uproariously together, we loved local dances we attended. There was then such intense positive energy there. This see-sawing I later discovered was a hallmark of abusive relationships.

All in all, however, I was living a lie and a very dangerous one for which I was to pay dearly in later years.

CHAPTER 8

Thrown Off The Roller Coaster

I have found it really hard to continue writing at this stage, perhaps a writer's block mirroring the huge emotional blocks that found me stuck in a highly dangerous situation, daily getting ground under and beginning to show signs of clinical depression. Still with no job, I was signing on on behalf of the family and had the regular ordeal of presenting myself at the Job Centre and applying for jobs that I was, as regularly, turned down for. I was over-qualified for them all. We lived precariously on dole money and undeclared earnings from Des's gardening, which were of course erratic due to Galloway's frequent rainy weather. He also insisted on having three months off in the winter to concentrate on his political work – he saw this as his right, not as the privilege of an upper-class man with a huge sense of entitlement and an exaggerated opinion of his own importance in the political scene.

At length the World Court Project reached the International Court of Justice in the Hague and in 1997 the court reached its inevitable conclusion. Des's team had laboured for years for no concrete improvement in the global security situation. He somehow managed to retrieve a sense of moral victory from this defeat. But worn down by our constant rows over his frequent absences from home, he decided to change the focus of his politics to local work. Instead of him being away every few weeks for a longish block, now he was out every second night. I had to struggle with him to spend time with Craig and myself.

Meanwhile I became involved in funding and starting a Rape Crisis Centre in Dumfries. This was taxing work and the team I was part of were definitely not feminists. However I felt I belonged to something worthwhile for a couple of years. Then this all blew up in my face when I managed to secure three years of funding for a paid worker and got turned down for the job in favour of a younger woman who supported our service being open also to men. This was due in part to the votes of other members of the collective who did not understand the importance of upholding the practise of the Rape Crisis network. It was also against our constitution and our very place in the Scottish network.

I put in an official complaint, not only to the centre but also to our funders. I was expelled summarily from the collective. It was a ghastly period. Not one of the collective supported me, though I found support from a local older feminist, formerly of Women's Aid who had in the same way been forced out of her job there after many years of dedicated input. I did put in a complaint to the Network which, after many agonizing months for me, took the Dumfries centre to task for what they had done. And though this was a moral victory, it was support from very far away and I felt very betrayed by other women in my locality and team.

Another person who stood by me in all this was Marion, who was the director of a local alcohol counselling agency. She had 'headhunted' me whilst I was with Rape Crisis and I went through the Scottish Council for Alcohol training with flying colours. From then on I did two or three counselling sessions per week. At first I found it really worrying as I took my clients' issues home. But eventually I got through that stage and did feel a sense of pride in what I was doing. However I felt a fraud underneath as my own life was based on the denial of the abuse that was being regularly inflicted on me.

This abuse took a dreadful toll on me when I was menopausal, triggering massive bleeding which reached haemorrhage point at one stage. I once was sent to hospital with so much bleeding that a miscarriage was suspected. We diligently and desperately continued with our 'therapy' which in retrospect was really crap and I was later badly betrayed by one of these 'therapists' when I went public about the abuse which she knew about. All in all, I was regularly being bruised badly, mainly on my upper legs, once Des jumped on my stomach, once he held me down and spat over my face, even though I pleaded with him to stop – this was the one and only occasion I showed any vulnerability in such sessions. I pleaded "Please let me up, I have been raped" but he continued. Once I had to have eight stitches in my hand as he pushed me over, I fell on a piece of glass and my hand was deeply cut. I was weeping in the car but he did nothing but scowl at me all through the ride to the hospital and when I was being stitched up. Another dreadful repeated scenario was when he shoved me bodily down the loft ladder. It was only luck that I somehow seemed to land safely, rather than breaking my neck.

Early on when the violence started I went to the police but I was in a state of utter panic as we were in the midst of a flaming row – we had been driving and were in the local town. I leapt out of the car, rushed into the police station and blurted out that my partner was being violent to me. Des however rushed in behind me and made the counter-accusation that I was hitting him and he was merely retaliating. We left the police station both having received a warning- this left me feeling that no help was possible from those paid to protect.

Another aspect to his abuse was his completely exposing my wounded-ness and then emotionally tormenting me. For example, I was not willing to stop at his command for men hitchhikers due to fear of unknown male passengers. One day we passed a local man it turns out we knew. Des's sensibilities were so smitten by guilt about it that he went to the man involved to explain - he told the guy that we had not stopped because I had been raped. I was furious that he had told this to a local village man. He asserted he had done nothing undermining of my needs and that I should be open about it. The row was so awful I rang my faithful friend, Shirley, who dropped everything and came driving the twelve or so miles to defend me. I also was regularly returning this support to her in her struggles with a similar chauvinist.

When Megan was about twenty-one, I became aware that she was still bulimic and there followed another horrible year which ended in my giving her an ultimatum - either she get hospital help or I would have to cut off from her. It seemed that Daniel was telling her the same. She did go for help and whilst she was on the NHS waiting-list, I paid for her to get more private therapy at £50 a session. Still to this day I do not know how effective this help was and to what extent my darling Megan still wrestles with this awful demon, probably now in the form of self-starvation, alternating with subsisting on fudge and chocolate accompanied by what seems to me a rather punishing exercise regime. She did wisely say at the time that she was only going for help for the sake of Daniel and myself and that this was not a good basis for therapy. But she then added that she did not want to lose us, so she supposed it was really for her own account that she was going.

Still unemployed, there was however another new community-project that occupied my time. The Scottish Executive financed a pilot programme in the regions of Scotland for funding of local projects. I completed the application-form on behalf of our village and we secured an award. The village then went through a community-needs assessment facilitated by two council workers and we formulated a village development plan. I put in another funding application which secured £25,000, enough money for us to buy a sizeable piece of land. The project was to include play-space, an orchard, a labyrinth and other features. For three years or so I worked hard on this committee. Des has been slightly involved at the start but backed off, probably because he could not be boss of the outfit. He tended to work only in situations where he was number one.

It was mostly very boring thankless work and I do not know how I endured it except I reckoned I might as well be doing something of use to the community whilst I was unemployed or unemployable. Moreover the Chair, Robert, was so dominating and sexist that our organisers told me that if I pulled out, they would probably cancel our funding, because otherwise the project would be scuppered by him and I was a key team-member in keeping the project on track. And in fact all the work our committee put into it bore great fruit in that the land is now permanently in community-ownership with a play space, a bar- B- Q space, a playground, a field, a labyrinth and many lovely trees.

Another community project I pulled off was more enjoyable and I was involved in it for nearly three years. That was a women's samba band for which I secured the funding, bought the equipment and hired the teacher. This took many hours of research on my part. Thus was born the Belties, which several years later still survives as two women's samba bands. What an enthusiastic racket we made and what a great laugh we had afterwards meeting in the pub. Round 1997, Wigtown had become designated and funded as a book-town and attracted a dynamic feminist called Karen. She was pretty key to our Belties social life. Many social events were held in her home next to her bookshop, Reading Lasses. This was a fun part of my life.

It was around 1997 also that Craig sat his Highers and sailed easily through them getting 5 A's. I had been very worried that he would not do well as his school years had been marked by very little work done at home. He decided to take a gap year and he went to stay with his Dad for the summer at Callum's home of the last few years in a community in Lancashire. He really liked being there as there were lads of his age to hang out with, and he stayed on after the summer, so effectively he left home in 1998 though that had not been the plan.

I missed him terribly but thought that perhaps Des and I could now stabilize without the frequent rows that surfaced over my alleged dreadful mothering. For a few month things rumbled on much as before. But again with hindsight it seems Des saw Craig's departure as an opportunity to leave me and his threats on this score increased, destabilising me further. At one point sex was painful due to menopausal dryness and I said semi-jocularly, "Thank God that's over." He then decided to withdraw from me even further and said he would sleep in Craig's bed. I asked him not to and he returned to our matrimonial bed. But he made no further sexual advances.

It was in November of 1998 that I got a phone call that sent me screaming into the living-room. Callum told me he had been diagnosed with skin cancer. I felt at once that this was going to be terminal. Des asked me what was wrong but I did not tell him. Callum did not want the kids to be told at this stage and I knew Des could never be trusted to keep a secret.

I cannot remember which year things happened but either then, or a year later, Delilah, the younger of our two spaniels, had nine puppies which sold and with the money, I paid for myself, Des and Craig to go on a group-adventure holiday in Morocco. This could have been wonderful but Des was really horrible to me all through it. I was moreover very nervous as we were awaiting on our return the results of further diagnostic tests for Callum. Des insisted on arguing unpleasantly with a man in our group who was a Pepsi Cola PR man and thus an easy target for Des's superior lectures about corporate shit. He wearied everyone with his sermons. Moreover he showed his true colours when I was felt up in his presence by an Arab – Des saw what happened but when I told him that I felt really demeaned, he raised no objection in my solidarity – instead he told me I must not cause a fuss and that in this country there was a different code on such matters. !!!

On our return we went straight to visit Callum. His news was bad. He had prostrate cancer level three. The kids had been told about the cancer by this time but they were not told now how bad things were. I had tried a few months previously to prepare them, they had both told me emphatically that, as usual, I was being pessimistic.

The next few months rolled by. I started to have insomnia and began to lose the extra stone I had gained during the menopause. I then lost a further stone and began to look like a rake. I started to have horrible racking pain in my buttocks and stomach with loose bowels, the start of years and years of what became non-stop acute pain I alleviated only by spells on an SSRI. I was examined by a Gastro- specialist in Edinburgh who found nothing clinical. My friends began to worry that I had anorexia. I was eventually sent to a psychiatrist who diagnosed severe clinical depression and I was assigned to a therapist called Laura. But it was not therapy I needed but affection, a cessation of the violence and stability in my life. That was not to happen.

As the millennium approached I remembered the thought I had had since I could count – that at the dawn of 2000 I would be 54 and I would be very old, my life nearly over. Now I had no idea what my life was about, except that I had to keep Des at any cost. All my traumas required me to keep him there, to win his love and make a happy ending, but after a lousy millennium celebration when he cold-shouldered me, on January 18th 2000, he left. He left on the day I had had to drive to attend the funeral of one of my alcohol clients - in the evening whilst I had been out at the Belties.

I now fell apart. When I saw the usual note left on the kitchen-table, my heart went into over-drive. I was gripped by the familiar terror of yet another runner. Another note about it all being over and blaming me. All the past occasions Des had left me, my only thought was to get him back. But something within me had changed. Six weeks before he had been telling me he was going to leave and I had said, "Please stop this, can't you see I am having to deal with Callum's impending death." He retorted coldly "Just how long after he is dead can I leave?" He was sadistically copying, word for word, the line that I had in trust confided in him, the line of Callum's about my father's death that had been accompanied by a kicking and that had finished that relationship for me. Now twelve years later the same words delivered to me but with a twist of added cruelty - I heard a voice in my head which said "Even I do not deserve this." And something like the realization that this was not a man who deserved my love.

So now all the night of his departure I lay awake on a rack having to get up every twenty minutes to empty my bowels which had turned to water. I do not know how I got through the next few years because this hell continued that long. The only thing I knew was that, this time, I was never to ask him to come back. I must never again put myself in the position of being tormented by him with his mocking and cold refusals and disdain for my abject state. Prompted by one of my friends, Shirley, I went again to the police and reported his violence. This time but too late, they took it seriously as I was able to take along several letters he had written to me talking explicitly about various acts of violence to me.

But Des was not going to take this lying down. On Feb 14th he sent out about a hundred letters, several of which were eight-pages long and full of sordid details. These letters basically denounced me and accused me of initiating the violence, then presented his long-suffering self as understandably "occasionally" losing it in response. The letters went to all my friends and to all the people we had any connection to at all, including to my siblings, the alcohol agency, and people in our village. It was horrific. What was worse was the number of my 'friends' who believed him or thought his smearing campaign was o.k.

To this day I have no idea who has read all this shit about me. Certainly from this point one of my closest friends, Grete , told me that wherever she went in the region, if she said she came from our village, folk said "Oh God, that is where that dreadful woman comes from " – referring to myself – this from people who did not even me know me in many cases.

I was in the meantime in an agony of missing Des. I could barely function. I felt unable to work as an alcohol counsellor and resigned. They had got the eight-pager about me and were disgusted with Des and supportive but I was in no fit state to work in such an arena.

I asked Des to meet with me and not to cut off from me. We met a few times but it was always with him being cruel and then he decided he would not continue as he said I was too emotional and in any case it might prejudice his case. But I had to see him pass on the street and hear about his doings from friends and read his right-on letters in the press. I replied to some of them, naming his conduct and in fact the Galloway News did print some of my replies. I felt driven to such a public airing by his prior cruel letter campaign.

Now imagine the brass-neck of the man. He had joined a group of very conservative Buddhists the previous year and now struck up a pose of a spiritual exemplar and mentor. But what crowned it all for me was to learn that he was offering classes on anti-sexism in the local school evening-classes, this while he still had criminal charges pending for violence to a local woman. This was too much for me. I found out when the class was being held, saw his car in the car-park and left a placard on it denouncing him for his violence. I also did this whilst he was sitting meditating in his Serene Reflection group. These actions I did on my own but they left me feeling a bit stronger.

Another horrible development. On speaking to Sylvie on the phone around 2001 she told me that she had attended a party in Bristol where a young woman remembered her from years back, when she had been close with her family. Des had apparently done childcare for her as a little girl aged around eleven or twelve and had scared her out of her wits by insisting she play the 'undressing game' with him and Eric. Apparently only Eric's intervention stopped Des. I asked Sylvie if she was not concerned for Eric, and she assured me not. This felt really wrong to me at the time and, several years later, more was revealed that threw further light into Sylvie's possible situation in all this. However back in 2001 I was then thrown into a dreadful dilemma.

At this point in Galloway here was a huge official vortex going on about possible sexual offences to children and vulnerable young adults centering on Kilquhanity alternative school, Lauriston alternative community and Samye Linghe Buddhist monastery. A horrible thought came into my mind and would not leave, fuelled by many remarks made by Sylvie and little things Des himself had said to me, including his confessing to running his hand up his daughter's leg when she was a   baby when he was 'not getting on with her mother'. So the question which took up residence in my mind was - to what extent had Des been involved in all this? I reported my concerns to the police dealing with my case. I stressed that I had questioned my children about this and they had reported that there had never been any crossing of boundaries with them by Des. Of course this got back to Des and he stepped up his propaganda campaign about how I was crazy and vindictive and this was the accepted community verdict about me in many minds.

It was many months before the Procurator Fiscal decided that he was going to drop the case. There was no evidence to corroborate mine. My neighbours, who had at least once witnessed Des dragging me out onto the road and kicking me, were not willing to give evidence. He had got away with it. I had suspected as much. He then tried to win some more brownie points, not by crowing - that would not have been as effective as his strategy - of weeping to people about how bad he felt that I had not got justice. But he did not ask of himself to show that his remorse was genuine and to go back to the police and plead guilty and I suspect none of his circle asked it of him. It was at this point that I discovered that he had started a new relationship.

Now I really was in agonies. The first few months had probably been ones where I had still had vestiges of hope that Des would recognize the error of his ways, go to therapy specifically for violent men, come back to me a new man and there would at last be a happy ending. I really still could not accept the reality of the situation – that Des was an abusive man. Moreover a highly dangerous man because of his upper-class use of propaganda, his charm offensive, impression-management and infiltration of all the networks which were important to me.

What made his new relationship more horrendous for me was that it was with a woman called Grace W, who was a counsellor who had been taken on by the local hospital, which was finding it hard to get properly trained therapists. This is where I was a patient. Grace W. knew this only too well and she knew that Des had been charged with violence towards me. Almost a year of hell followed, as I put in an NHS complaint. My complaint was tossed back by the Health Board and was eventually referred to the Mental Health Commission where, after months of endless letters and being in an agony of suspense, it was eventually upheld. Meanwhile I had to get therapy elsewhere.

Also whilst all this was going on, in 2001, Callum's life began to come to a close. Craig was only twenty and in the midst of his university studies. Moreover his Dad's new partner, Rhona, was very territorial and did not want me to be involved at all in his care. She really messed me about and earned the anger of Callum's community. One time just before the end I took the kids down to see Callum. As well as driving such a long distance, from Galloway to Edinburgh then to Lancs then back, Rhona required that I cook dinner for the community on arrival. But we were hit by a car, luckily in a slow-moving queue and the car I had borrowed was written off. Craig had been huddled in the back sleeping off a hang-over and was showered in broken glass. He could have been killed. No sympathy from Rhona.

I had the most horrendous thirty-six hours when the end came. I had just completed the round trip down with the kids when there was a phone call from Rhona to say the end was soon and to come straightaway. I leapt back into the car and drove in the dark to Edinburgh to pick up an exhausted Craig. Megan decided not to come and later I was glad as I think Rhona would have had her banned from Callum's presence too. As that was what she did to me. I was not allowed to go into Callum's deathbed and was told by Rhona that Callum did not want me there.

Callum's housemates told me later that Rhona had been taking it upon herself to select who could see Callum and misrepresenting it as Callum's wishes. The people she excluded were mainly women and people who had a close link with Callum. Anyway she ignored the understandable need of Craig to have his mother with him as he sat through his father's dying. But neither Craig or I wanted an argument in front of a dying Callum, so I chose to sit nearby in an adjacent relatives' room. A couple of hours later in the middle of the night, I heard the sound of Callum's last breath. For a couple of hours I held a shaking and weeping son. My heart was really stretched to its limit.

From then on Craig put his grief behind him. He had to go back to the demands of a University course, which he completed, and did well two years later. How proud Callum would have been to see his son walk up to get his degree. And my heart was really sore as I watched Craig's broad shoulders swing up the long aisle to receive his degree. I was sitting by myself, my heart aching to share the joy and pride with Callum. And Megan and Daniel were unavoidably late for the ceremony and could not get a seat near me. Anyway that was away down the line.

The funeral gave me a chance to reclaim a proper place in the life of Callum, though Megan and I were not selected to bear the coffin – this was done chiefly by Rhona's friends and Craig. But I did give a tribute to Callum which publicly honoured the strength of our connection. I honestly do not know how I managed to get through all this. At one point I was driving down to Lancashire and an elderly friend was kindly following me in his car. I was so drugged by Valium that I began to zone out. He noticed that I had started to weave over the road and he attracted my flagging attention by hooting. It took two cups of black coffee to wake me up enough to drive safely. Also after the funeral I trusted this friend to drive Craig and his friend to catch a train but I did not find out till later that he was driving at 70 m.p.h. drunk and stoned. How close to the wind I was sailing.

Back in Galloway I was being held together by anti-depressants and managed to stagger through each day spending a lot of time firing off letters to the various groups in which Des and Grace postured as right-on alternative stars. I publicly and repeatedly requested that the members of these groups require these stalwarts of right-on-ness to attend mediation with me to improve the situation, or even to try to persuade Des to have the decency to attend Callum's funeral to support Craig. He told one of my friends that he thought I was lying about Callum's health to enlist sympathy. What a bastard! This was only a few days before Callum's death and I was desperate for some care and support.

Moreover his Buddhist women friends made my life even more difficult. One of them, a real nasty piece of work called Jessica, was in the Belties. After I had secured yet another grant to keep the group going, one might have thought I would get a pat on the back or some gesture of appreciation from her. But Jessica saw fit, in our group-meeting, to quibble about 40p worth of photocopying that she claimed I could have got cheaper elsewhere. I expressed anger about this- there was no apology, I said I had had enough of the dynamics in the group around her, which had been apparent to all for some time – she stood next to me and beat out the rhythm all wrong as loud as she could. When I tried to politely question it, she insisted she had got it right. Moreover, when I had tried to raise it,

I was made out by some group members to be dumping on Jessica because she was an ally of Des. The rest stayed silent. I asked for an apology from Jessica about quibbling about 10p and of course none was forthcoming. When I tried to speak calmly to her on the street about it, she went straight into vindictiveness. She said she would call the police, a tactic obviously recommended by Des to deal with this "mad woman". She then misrepresented me to others.

I got no support from anyone else in the Belties and I left the only group that had been fun for me and one that I had funded. Some couple of years later my issue about her drumming was vindicated, it seems the teacher was all too aware of the problem of Jessica's errant rhythm - but because she stopped over at Jessica's, she felt she could not pull her up on it. So I had been made the scapegoat due to women's unwillingness to engage in conflict –resolution or basic honesty.

The only positive project in my life for those next two years was the community labyrinth which I worked on laboriously on my own, day after day, shifting heavy wheel-barrows of pebbles for the path, in all weathers, and foraging for wild flowers. I had a few loyal friends and soon came to know who they were. My menopause group, which I had started a few years back, was still going and they were all loyal to me apart from two of the Buddhists who eventually dropped out, though for other reasons. The three stalwarts are still my true friends to this day. Another friend of mine started a meditation group in the village and this was another weekly haven. I also had a lovely new friend in the village, Grete, who was going through a messy separation and had a wild child, and I really loved both of them.

One day whilst I was toiling away on the labyrinth I had a sudden flash. I was to move up north and re-connect with Findhorn. At the time this seemed crazy as my last connection there had been one of open public dissidence and I knew I would not be welcome by some of the old guard. But over the next fortnight, two things happened to confirm this next step. One was the sudden receipt of a Findhorn brochure out of the blue- it was personally addressed to myself and Megan. The other was a reference by someone completely unexpected. I decided to brave it and booked to go on the 40th birthday week.

This marked the beginning of my second Saturn return, the next phase of my life where at last I begin to break away from the nexus of abuse, to try to break my ties to a perpetrator and to leave an area where my name had become mud in the mouths of many.

CHAPTER 9

Mending My Life

The months dragged by with more of the same and my plans to move firming up. They were made even more urgent by another horrible development. I discovered that Des had left Galloway with Grace to join a community in Fife. He told people he had to leave because he was scared to go out anywhere in the region in case he banged into me.

The community was home to several young kids and I thought some dope-smoking, a combination I reckoned would possibly knock out Des's controls in relation to children. So, after consulting a child-abuse expert, I contacted the community and the local social work department about Des's lack of sexual and other boundaries with kids. This got back to Des who dragged all his friends into it, making out that I was insane, beyond reason and merely on a vicious vendetta. He even talked with them about taking legal action against me which I discovered years later. This must have been empty posturing - it allowed him to declare that he had nobly decided not to go down the legal route out of concern for the fact that I was clearly insane and all this would damage Craig.

However he felt no compunction about involving Craig himself, dragging him into it on his side. I then had the awful task of listening to my son in a distraught state accusing me of a vendetta. And I felt really split in two as I knew that it was important for Craig to have some sense of a decent father-figure in

Des. So I told him merely that I had this information from Sylvie. Craig dismissed this as ranting by a horrible woman which should not be credited. I said nothing more to answer this to preserve Craig's state of mind.

But Craig was terribly upset with me – in the end he understood that my concerns were sincere and not vengeful but Des and Grace were required to leave their new home following on my letter. I also lost a friend over this, Marion, who thought I was just being vindictive. Really I suspect she was upset because one of her friends had been in trouble over leaks of stuff re my NHS complaint. Anyway it was all horrible but I must admit that I felt a great sense of vindication that Des had not been able to start a new life free of even a slight bit of the baggage he had dumped on me. It appears that his new housemates were shocked that he had not breathed a word to them about all his troubles with me. And years later, after his death, more concrete details came out about Des's possible abuse of Eric that really vindicated what I had done. I had a conversation with a woman to whom Eric had allegedly confided the full nasty story - and I also heard accounts from other sources

Back to my own plans to move. I put my house on the market and it was bought straightaway over the internet at what seemed the princely sum of £75k – this for a cottage in a bad state of repair. I had two months to find somewhere near Findhorn and did it. Forres seemed out, on grounds of aesthetics, Findhorn was too expensive but in Burghead I saw a cottage with potential. It reminded me of my Grandma's cottage, which is what clinched it for me. Also I went for a walk with a childhood friend, David, along the headland with its rugged peninsula and staggering views across the Moray Firth. I knew this was it. For years I had been dreaming repeatedly about a beautiful sunny sea-shore with waves breaking in the sun-shine. If I looked from Burghead towards Hopeman, this could have been the shore of my dream. My offer was over-high and it was accepted. I was due to move in on Beltaine 2003.

I had begun to clear the house months before but now it proceeded in earnest. It was very harrowing deciding which items of my children's past and our joint lives together to throw out. Megan made one of her rare visits to Galloway, not to support me through the hard times, which she really could not seem to handle- but really to collect some items like the piano and dresser.

And as the time came near, I held a farewell gathering in the local town for all my women friends and that went o.k. – I tried hard not to be affected by the missing faces of those who had defected to Des's camp. Then the village held a farewell-event for me in gratitude for all I had done for the community. There was a marquee up in the field whose purchase I had funded. So it was held in there. There was a big turn-out and a speech of tribute and I did feel appreciated, though only close to my two friends in the village,

And it was Grete, not my kids, who helped me move house. I got hold of a cheap removal-van and drove up with two dogs and three cats. And Grete followed with her seven-year old son, Billy. We arrived in Burghead about six in the evening and of course there were no beds and the basics were all in boxes.

But we got something together. It was such an act of friendship from Grete as she was already having huge stresses in her own life. I will always be indebted to her and her loyalty in the face of all the horrid stories that were being fed to her about me.

Then she had to set off back south and I began my new life. I was buoyed up for a few days then suddenly reality hit. I was really low. There was lots of work needed to get the cottage in shape and I set about getting that done, spending quite a lot of my capital on updating the decor. All this took about four months. Building up a new friendship network took much longer. But, from where I am now, I have to give myself credit for what I achieved on all fronts over the next few years. My childhood and my repeated re-enactments since, culminating in the dreadful denouement with Des, had brought all my suppressed trauma up for me to deal with and my health was acutely bad, both emotionally and physically. I had IBS, clinical depression and complex PTSD which really needed specialized care. This was not available. And I went on a search for proper professional care from one expensive therapist to another, many of them hopelessly bad and two re-traumatising NHS therapy-groups which were only short-lived.

For many years life was mostly dominated by huge pain and suicide was a frequent yearning that I did not have the luxury to consider. It was something I had ruled out much earlier in my life, knowing the impact it would have on those who care for me. So I was trapped for many years in an agonizing and wretched world of emotional hell and serious bodily pain – this I had to cover up from most people in order to cope with life and to build a new network.

But I do have a strong fighting-spirit and I applied this as well to meeting people. I joined all sorts of groups, many associated with the Findhorn spiritual community, but I also started two in Burghead, one a meditation group and another one, a book group. I had moved to the town thinking it would be a provisional base until I managed to get into a co-housing community. But there was not one in existence so I got together with others to form what became a Cohousing coop which tried over many years to get a site at, or near to, Findhorn.

The meetings were long and were yet another situation of detailed complex documents, not a load of fun. But I did find excitement in Franco Santoro's astro-shamanic group which I belonged to for nearly two years. I was also part of a Non Violent Communication group, but what became a regular place of meditation and support for me was a Zen group in the tradition of Tchich Nhat Hahn which meets every Saturday morning with the wonderful practise of sharing from the heart and deep listening. I however did not find Buddhist teachings at all compatible with the earth–based ways that remain my core practise and the mainstay of my precarious health.

The children came to see me, Megan, once after I moved in and Craig regularly at Christmas and usually in the summer. His life progressed and in spite of all this grief and worries, he got a good degree and went to Newcastle to do a Ph D., which, after two years of hard work, he secured whilst holding down a job and writing up the thesis at night. He moved back to

Edinburgh. There were many hard issues for him to deal with, in particular being dumped after each major loss but I anticipate slightly here. Let me just say here that for a while, after I moved North, I did not have to worry too much about Craig.

But on my natal family-front, problems arose again. In 1999 Margaret had been admitted to mental hospital in Malta where she lived and she became progressively more ill. Her depression was aggravated by huge doses of drugs, ECT and a lousy marriage. Eventually she wanted to come back to the UK. She had already tried a few suicide-bids and, on a visit to Elizabeth tried again, which Elizabeth, in an already fragile state, found hard to deal with. She had just had to retire from her social work job, worn down by bullying. She was in an alarming state of health, both psychologically and physically. Moreover she had spent her money wildly and she got into debt. I had bailed her out twice. All this worry about Margaret pushed her further down.

Meanwhile I tried to get on with my life the best I could. I had never been close to Margaret, especially after the death of mum when she really laid into myself and Ewan. But it was a worry for me that I could do nothing but ring her.

My friendships were rather erratic as folk associated with Findhorn tended to be here today, gone tomorrow. And I was still drawn too easily into dysfunctional relationships. After an abortive attempt at a relationship with a man much younger than myself with what turned out to be a serious drug-problem - he died - I started attending 12-step programmes to do with my co-dependency. NHS therapy was pretty disastrous and I will not elaborate on the absolute outrageous way I was mis-treated by one therapist in a NHS group, when I tried to challenge a member about exposing her daughter to a man on parole from prison on child porn offences.

By this time I was having to deal with my attraction to abusive connections even more face-on as I had resumed contact with Des, whom I had glimpsed from a few feet away at the anti-G8 gathering in Stirling. This had been a tremendously empowering camp for me to attend and I was especially happy to be in a barrio that included Starhawk and to be on a convoy with her, blocking delegates on the A9 from reaching Gleneagles and being chased by the police. I saw Des, looking very Rasuptin-like, with an ominous umkempt grizzled beard, distributing leaflets as was his wont. I also found piles of 9/11 DVD's which he had bought for free distribution. I e-mailed him to say I was involved in 9/11 stuff. He could not then resist bombarding me with his output on that topic and gradually our correspondence became more personal.

I asked him to meet up with me so that we could reach a modus vivendi where we could at least attend family events like Craig's Ph D ceremony together. But he resisted, I think mainly out of fear and because Grace outlawed it. His relationship with her was still very on-and-off and she in fact left him to go and live in Nepal. She changed her mind after a year and came back. But no sooner had she left these shores, than he consented to see me. He looked dreadful when we met at the Culdees bunkhouse in the Trossachs on the banks of Loch Tay. I was alarmed by the fact that his health was clearly very bad, as he could only walk a short distance before his breathing became a bit laboured. I immediately suspected serious heart problems. On the emotional front I was still very much in love with him and had to put up with his still blaming me for my alleged 'mistreatment of poor Grace.' We agreed to leave that matter aside. I asked him eventually to promise not to end our connection if Grace came back. Des stuck to that in spite of the fact that it later caused continual struggle between himself and Grace.

In fact he started to offer me practical support. He would help me with driving to visit the kids, as I found negotiating the Edinburgh ring-road overwhelming in my emotional state. Then the dreadful news came that Margaret had died. Ewan had tried to help her by offering her support to return to the UK and she came to Devon where he lived for assessment by the NHS. She was in hospital briefly, then was told she was not allowed to stay there longer. The staff wanted her to return to Malta but she landed up with no alternative but a nursing-home, slowly declining, with no life and no contact outside the home apart from Ewan and his family. The nursing-home was not empowered to keep its clientele on suicide-observation and she started to save pills for another suicide attempt. However her life soon ended after what seemed like a deliberate fall down a set of stairs and two days of painfully slow dying.

The funeral was rife with distress. There was terrible tension between Elizabeth and Margaret's husband, Eddy and the finale of a huge public row in a pub between Ewan and his ex wife – she loudly blamed Ewan for Margaret's death. What a family! - I came home crushed. At that point Des was very supportive by e-mail and gave me £1,000 towards the costs of all the family-trips.   In fact I repaid him after Margaret left me a quarter of her estate which amounted to   £10,000 for myself.

Then came a dreadful row with Megan. She was toiling with the strain of not being able to conceive, undergoing the rigours of IVF, working long hours as deputy manager of a nursery, travelling daily to Edinburgh from the Borders where she and Daniel had moved and on top of that doing an Open University degree.   Anyway, I was also overwrought just a few weeks after Margaret's death and on a visit to Megan, we quarrelled over the trivial fact that I turned down the offer of a meringue. It was utterly devastating as afterwards, I asked her to make me a cup of tea I was so shaken. She refused, saying I had always asked her to bail me out. I lost my temper and demanded to know what I had done to raise such a callous daughter. I also asked her how she would feel right after the death of her brother. She was outraged, querying how I could say such a thing to her.

The full nasty repercussions really hit a few months later when, on my next visit, Daniel flew at me because I was allegedly being rude by choosing to leave the TV room where whole evenings went by without either of them barely talking to me - certainly that was Daniel's style but even Megan made little effort to make me feel part of the company. They would chat to each other whilst watching TV programmes to which I could not relate. So I had gone through to the kitchen, feeling humiliated and trying to distract myself by catching up on e-mails. Daniel let me have a load of abuse.

I was horrified at what was happening as Megan was at this point about six months pregnant and with twins. Towards the start of the row, Daniel was slagging me off as a dreadful mother. I appealed to Megan for support but she said that she did not want to take sides. Eventually I let loose with counter-accusations of macho behaviour.

I decided I had to create a boundary to protect myself and told Megan that if Daniel ever spoke to me like that again, I would leave and never come back. His response was to cold-shoulder me from then on.

On my next visit I was to stay in a Bed and Breakfast but then was allowed back into the home after a couple of such visits. What upset me most was not the fact that I could not fully enjoy the wonderful little boys who were eventually born but that it seemed to me that Daniel's treatment of myself indicated a complete disregard as to how this must really hurt Megan and later on his own sons who came to love me. I could not bear what he was doing to my daughter.

I also felt anguish for Megan who was 'choosing' to live with a man with such a capacity to sulk. For many years I awaited an improvement on this front but none was forthcoming, this in spite of the fact that in 2010, I bailed Daniel out financially, when his own father, who clearly was better-off than me , would not.

Next back to matters with Des. Our increasing rapprochement eventually came to a head in 2009. He had visited me once with Craig to help move a lot of Craig's stuff for storage at my cottage. And I had visited him several times in the poky little damp flat he rented in Perth where I was consigned to a cupboard-like bedroom on my own. Des was always at pains to let me know that he was 'in love with' Grace, until it became clearer in 2008, as their relationship deteriorated, that he would have to choose between us . In early 2009 he chose me.

But by then, the man I was still hopelessly in love with was in a parlous state indeed. In fact, I thought he had Parkinson's as well as heart disease. His short-term memory was failing rapidly. He visited me several times, we shared the same bed, he started to become integrated into my new life, to attend Findhorn events with me, to walk in Speyside in the spring. This was not a time of undiluted joy, however, for two reasons. Des kept having bouts of openly hankering after Grace and playing me off against her. He started to drive me frantic with anguish by insisting that he wanted to have the right to sex with her - even though he seemed incapable of having sex with anyone at this time. In retrospect it seems to me that Des had, some of the time, lost touch with what was actually happening.

I became very fraught all the time as the chronic triangle now seemed to have become acute. Moreover I was desperately worried about his health and convinced that he was seriously ill. I was also shocked that nobody else in his life seemed to have noticed, particularly Grace. I nagged him to go for medical checks which he duly did. But they all came back negative. I never-the-less kept at him to ask for more checks and wrote a letter to his doctor saying I thought he needed further urgent investigation. All to no avail.

Tests did not happen in time.   On a few occasions he referred to having been attacked whilst in a white van and had his head messed with.

Then finally on a visit to him I found him seriously ill, with virtually no short-term memory but talking a lot of having just visited Grace which floored me and also more talk of the white van attack. I took him straight to emergency care and he was admitted to a psychiatric hospital.

He was treated with anti-psychotic medication, never properly diagnosed and died suddenly three weeks later in the middle of the night. Even though I had sensed he was dangerously ill, his death was a huge shock to me. It   was later officially declared to be due to heart failure caused by limbic encephalitis. The subsequent autopsy found no cause for this condition and this, coupled with the claims he had made to me about having been attacked whilst in a van and had his head messed with, fuelled speculation among myself and his colleagues that he had been assassinated for his role in exposing state terrorism.

The next year I reacted by immersing myself in a struggle to get the authorities to investigate if there was anything more sinister about Des's illness. Many of his colleagues and I spent hours on the phone and writing letters, ringing the hospital, seeing lawyers and trying to get records. There had been internet reports of devices which can cause the very central nervous system problems Des died of and others that could induce heart attacks. The immediate cause of Des's death was a heart attack though this was related to his brain swelling.

In all this I was also having to deal with his horrid family, in particular his particularly obnoxious sister, Enid. She had begun to loathe me immediately my relationship with Des evidenced problems many years ago, this in spite of the fact that she also found him difficult. And my accusations about his abuse of myself and possibly children made her worse. As I was not married to Des, I had no say over his care in hospital when he was out-of-it and Enid took over in a mega way. She relished the petty authority this gave here. Des's funeral arrangements were also her work. Although the family did organise an interfaith but mainly Buddhist event, there was no wake after for mourners to gather and share their feelings over Des – all in all, a mean affair. She even went so far as to hector me to move a bucket and mop as if I were a mere chamber-maid and she treated those of Des's colleagues who regarded his death as suspicious with equal disdain and coldness.

When she was settling his debts she delighted in telling me this willingness on the part of the family did not extend to sums he owed me - at the least £120, but she   hastened to sort out all debts to others. What a bitch!!

And then at the funeral, Robyn started telling me of problems that had arisen around Sylvie and her son, Eric. She, whilst dying of cancer around 2002, had allegedly confessed to a friend that she felt terrible guilt about ignoring sexual abuse of Eric by Des. Then Robyn told me more – that Sylvie's funeral was disrupted by a serious incident. This centred around a young woman who attended, spotted Des and became very distraught. She told older women there that she had to leave and she cited abuse of herself and Eric by Des as the reason. She could not be persuaded to stay. Women organising the funeral had debated asking Des to leave but the young woman left before they took action. A meeting was held afterwards where it was all discussed.

Robyn gave me the phone number and e-mails of two women who, she said, could give me more details. One would not answer my queries and we suspected that this was because we had the impression that Sylvie had indeed been complicit in the abuse of Eric and that this friend feared Sylvie's reputation as a feminist would suffer if this became public. Moreover, given the prominent position of both Sylvie and Des in the feminist community, such bad press would inevitably tarnish the feminist cause. However the silence of this woman to me as a mother concerned over possible abuse of my own children suggested to me that there was an issue here - as otherwise she could easily have put me out of my misery with an account which exonerated Des.

The other woman I did speak to on the phone for at least an hour. She told me explicitly that Eric had come to her in distress – she lived next door to Sylvie and family – she said he was distraught because Des had molested him by masturbation. She said there were several such incidents and that she eventually confronted Des. He flew into a rage and said it was none of her business. She also said that she had talked to Sylvie about it, suggesting she take Eric for medical examination. She said she got the impression that Sylvie was already aware of the situation but was not able to cope with it. She also thought Sylvie was too enmeshed with Des to see things straight. The amount of detail told me in this account had a certain ring of truth about it and I could think of no reason why this woman would lie though I did later find out that she had on occasions been known to fabricate things. However the allegations had also come from other quarters.

For Robyn also felt Des was 'guilty' and she cited his involvement in support (or as an active member, I was not sure) of the Paedophile Information Exchange which was a cause celebre of some alternative men of the late 70's. Their line was that children had right to sex with adults!!!. All in all, I could just imagine Des in the midst of such controversy, particularly as, at that time, anything went in his bohemian lifestyle with Sylvie. What a sordid mess.

I was horrified and though I could never get confirmation of any of this, I could no longer visit Des's grave in the beautiful green woodland site near Comrie. My grief was complicated enough as it was by all the confusion in his dealings between myself and Grace, some of which may have been due to his illness.

Des's death ended a chapter in my life or should I say three chapters in my life, as I had been connected to him for nearly twenty-one years, had loved him to distraction, lost him once, then finally lost him to a very problematic death shrouded in intrigue and subsequently even more complicated by allegations of his possible sexual misconduct.

My only consolation in all this was that I was the last person to speak to him before his death. His final words to me were "Gale. I am sorry I treated you badly." I replied "That's all right, you know I love you" to which he replied, rather forcedly "I love you too." The exchange felt coming from a deep soul level, however, and these were our final words to each other. Later I saw it as the angel of death brushing us with her wings. Moreover during his funeral ceremony, I noticed a plaque for the grave right next to his. I scraped the earth off to it to read the name and was really jolted when I read the name "Gale".

I was now 63 and had the chance to be finally free of this emotional mess and all that it stood for in terms of traumatic re-enactment. I really needed at last to get a life free of this sort of extreme instability. Since then I have been given another chance. My close friendships sadly still carry the scars. I still get drawn to women friends who are bright, engaging but prone to bouts of aggression. I have made a determined effort to heal from all this and to build a new life free from situations of tormenting relationships and to face myself on my own with no saviour. In fact I have not been able to fall in love since Des's death and now live in hope that secure love and hope can take root in my life and eventually flourish. This is an ambitious aim but I do have courage and tenacity. I live daily with the struggle against my depression and physical pain and the determination to live the life I have left as best I can, in spite of it all.

And my aim in writing this undeniably sad life-story is to give voice to my hunger to speak out for radical change in the way people who have been abused and highly traumatised are treated in a society at present wedded to traumatic social re-enactment.

This has been a hard tale to live and tell but I have written it to deliver an essential message. The NHS failed myself, all members of my family and those many others who have suffered serious abuse or trauma as dependent children. It still does on a daily basis. We are the most wretched and wounded of patients yet whilst treatment is quite rightly offered for OCD, depression, anxiety and the like, we, who are the most in need, are almost all offered nothing but drugs and short–term ineffective therapy. We are often given humiliating labels such as Borderline Personality Disorder, not another less stigmatising label such as Complex Post Traumatic Stress Disorder. The BPD patient e.g. is diagnosed as untreatable and thus written off. There are precious few staff trained in the treatment of childhood trauma and budgets do not allow the long-term treatment needed for recovery. Only those with resources can access properly designed private treatment.

The fact that I am alive today is not down to the NHS. In fact I have been seriously damaged by its faulty diagnoses and inappropriate treatments, grossly dangerous drugs and being fobbed off with cheap inappropriate options like CBT or Mindfulness. Putting all my energy into working at these options and then meeting with no improvement served only to further demoralise me and increase my sense of failure and inadequacy.

My survival is in large part due to the few brave individuals who have really helped me – they have often suffered the same sort of abuse as I have and have trained to help others but have to work privately – also to a couple of social workers who treated me as a human being, not as a patient-number or diagnostic label, to volunteers who extended me child-care support and the loving friendship of a few faithful compassionate friends- to my drive to expose the knowing abandonment of society which has written us off and offered us no safe haven to recover - and finally I am alive because of a feminist understanding of the roots of our collective misery and my determination not to succumb.

SWEET SISTER OF SORROW

This is the hardest story I will ever write. For in the writing I must weigh each detail, select each fragment, and turn it over to my inward gaze, include or discard, to reach a rare economy, where I know I have captured for myself the essentials of your life and death. In so doing, I hope I will build myself a monument to you and to the preciousness of your life. The task feels beyond me but somewhere and somehow I must begin.

Rosie, you were always ahead of me on life's path, your compact big sister's body astride my little world, your hand holding mine as I toddled, your finger guiding my eyes over my first reading book. I lived in wonder of you, you seemed so charged with life, your smile turned on the lights in my world. Your jet black hair framed a perfectly beautiful face with unforgettably blue eyes. With you I capered in forbidden glee, bouncing on our ancient bed in high jinx till our father burst through the door in a rage. Put to bed too early, we spent hours in mirth concocting stories about our stuffy neighbours, long sagas in which their respectable facades were ripped off by some ribald detail we had embroidered into their colourless lives. The coldly disapproving neighbour next door, Nosy Parker Roy, who was always tattling on our childhood pranks, we mated with the butcher in a crude frenzied orgy on the steps of her immaculate garden. She tossed her soiled knickers in the faces of the horror-stricken but riveted passersby. In our world we engineered the public disgrace of our hideous Headmaster, exposed to Her Majesty's School

Inspectorate for cheating to make his own school excel. You created a funfair world in which we rollicked for hours on end. Our childhood landscape you imbued with a magical nimbus. And it was you who revealed to me the true identity of the ominous block of rock that resided next to the old blacksmith's forge.

From you I learnt to write stories, and though you never lived to write your own, I hope what your life taught me can speak something of you. Your emotional life was irrepressible and infectious. You were not taken in by poppycock and you taught me how to laugh. You also unknowingly tried to teach me to cry, though that lesson was much harder. You held my body next to yours through many a stormy night. In my treasure-box of childhood memories I have two priceless pictures of you, both in the snow, when the frost had changed the blue-black of your shiny hair into a silvery hard filigree. You laughed so loud as the snow twirled about your radiant face. And, as always, your happiness made me so happy. You truly took me to the end of the rainbow and there was always a crock of gold there.

We lived together through a childhood of emotional and physical tyranny, cruelty and coldness, teetering ever on the brink of the next violent parental outburst. Violence to you put me off the violin - you showed me my bow that our father had broken on your back. Yet you strove bravely on. You forged ahead of me into secondary school. You tried to make sense of those tormented teenage trials. And I tagged along behind you. I watched you stand up to the might of our father.

And you alone of all the children in my world dared to defy bullies. You dared to wade into a crowd of older boys bullying an orphan, boys older than yourself. And your passionate outburst made them stop.

Of course, there were sore places between us, as between all sisters and brothers, however close. My nose streamed crimson blood over my pristine school blouse from the punch you delivered during a fight over a coveted toy. You sometimes teased me, enticing me to view some new treasure, only to deliver me a swipe on the face. At times your spontaneous sparkle embarrassed me in public, and I didn't like you singing as we trudged up the brae from school - what if some of our hidebound community thought we were weird?

Then there was the Christmas Day ruined for me because you had been promised a new bike all of your own. And in the end you were given one to share with me. When it was my turn to ride it that wintry afternoon, I set off down the road with these words ringing in my ears - "Keep the bike. I don't want it. You always spoil things for me." You never again rode our bike and your blaming accusation pinioned me helplessly to a cross of guilt for your pain and condemned me beforehand with a sense of total responsibility for your death. Yet, for the most part, in spite of the cruelty we were living with, you wove a vibrant life-filled world for me to share with you.

But then, as you started to enter womanhood and to bleed, your steps began to falter. You started to weep a lot. It seems as if your bleeding brought with it raw emotional outpourings of the torment of living in our unbearable family, imprisoned in a coldly violent school obsessed with good marks, and embedded in a Calvinist tomb of a community whose chief principle seemed to be to stamp out any joie de vivre in its young. I watched you nightly burst into tears as you struggled with mathematical hieroglyphics you couldn't fathom, impossible tasks required from you by stony-faced men with no appreciation that your gifts lay elsewhere.

You began to say that you hated yourself, that you were ugly, you were useless. You were true to yourself, you spoke your feelings and I couldn't stand them. I armoured myself against you. I began to feel condescending towards you. My sister was weak, and I could no longer be proud of you. Yet I did my best to boost you up with further servings of our tall stories. This time, they only worked for brief moments. Finally, a couple of years later, when you finally left home, you broke down altogether.

The done thing was done. You were sent to a Victorian mental hospital, a seventeen year old young woman overcome by the despair of trying to survive. 'Kindly' male doctors sadistically gave you the label 'hysteric', to trivialize and distance themselves from your pain and its <u>obvious</u> causes. They pumped you full of drugs that made you flop around the house on your rare visits home, that is when you weren't too sedated to get up. Recently a doctor at the hospital you were in told me that, nowadays, you would have been diagnosed as suffering from 'melancholia' - hence all the sedation you received in the 1960's undoubtedly depressed you further. They also injected you with insulin to convulse you out of your agony. In occupational therapy your numbed fingers made baskets and knitted misshapen jumpers nobody would ever wear. You plummeted down further and further during your two and a half years of 'treatment'. You swallowed a fork and other sharp objects to hurt yourself. You cut your arms with anything you could improvise as a weapon against yourself. You took more than the prescribed dose of barbiturates.

I saw you infrequently during those times, never in the hospital which we were forbidden to mention. And when, on your visits home, I left you to go to school, I would never know whether I would return to find you had once again been whisked off to hospital. All through this we, your sisters and brother, were to breathe not a word to anybody about your whereabouts and problems, this silence in spite of the fact that I would come home from school to perform such a harrowing task as lift your slumped body from the floor, your hands all bleeding from cuts caused by smashing some of our mother's ornaments; this silence in the face of my glimpses of your freshly cut arms, or the operation-scars on your stomach. You and your suffering were not to exist.

And so I suppose it was logical that you took your next and final successful step, one which I have tried to cancel out in my mind over and over. You had asked to be readmitted to hospital so you could live there and work outside. Somehow you landed up in the nightmare ward. You pleaded with our father to get you out. That shows me how desperate you must have been - to prefer our hell-hole of a family. Our father tried to get you out but our mother wouldn't let you come home. It was she who took the burden of your daily care, who tried to block the way between you and the death you so clearly desired. The hospital did not transfer you to an easier ward until a couple of weeks had passed. It seemed a shortage of beds confined you to a place from which you had clearly begged to be removed. In the new ward there were people your own age and you could work in the garden if you felt like it. I wonder if you felt like it in the last few days you had left, drugged to the eyeballs as you were.

On Good Friday our mother and father visited you. They took you for a walk on the seashore and to a restaurant for afternoon tea. Then our father asked if you wanted to come home for Easter. No, you told him, you were frightened of him. He became very upset at this and his upset really upset you.

The next day, in the late afternoon, you went missing when you were supposed to be gathering for tea with the others. A search was instituted. Your death report states you died by hanging. But in between these last two sentences opens up a whole world for me.

The bald facts, as far as I managed to piece them together years later, are that you went into a toilet, took off your dressing gown, made a noose out of the sleeves and clambered up by the toilet door. Somehow you managed to hang yourself over the toilet door. A young nurse found you a while later. Your face was pallid, your lips cyanosed. She rushed for the Duty doctor, Doctor A. They couldn't get you down easily as your body was blocking the toilet door. The doctor climbed up the partition and began hacking at your dressing gown with his scissors. The fabric tore and your body fell gently to the ground. The toilet door was opened.

'The patient's neck was freed from the garment and she was taken out into the corridor anteroom. Mouth to mouth breathing and external cardiac massage was initiated. After several minutes there was no colour change and these efforts were abandoned. No pulse, heart beat or sign of spontaneous respiration was found.'

You were dead.

'Dr A then informed Dr B who was on second call. Dr X the Deputy Physician Superintendant was also informed. The Procurator Fiscal and the City Police were informed and the body was removed to Lodge Walk for examination. Death was certified as being due to hanging. Dr X gave the death certificate.'

Your parents were assured that the death was instantaneous. Very few people saw you buried. None of your friends were there. Your sisters and brother were not allowed to go to the funeral. Worse, we never saw your body and we were not told what had happened to you, only that you had died. It was years later before I began to unearth the few details I have of your death and the last period of your life. It has taken me the rest of my life to retrieve your body for myself, to wash it with a sister's tears, to mourn for you and to release you. For so long, I tarred your death with the brush 'Cowards Way Out', prolonging my contempt for the depth of your expressed despair. I hated you for what I felt you had done to me and our family, stigmatising us as outcasts with an unmentionable secret. What chasms in myself did I hate so much as to consign you to my version of the Christian Hell reserved for the likes of you, to such unhallowed psychic ground?

A lot of the time for the first few years, I numbed you out, I pretended you had never been in my life. A lot of the time I was glad you, or at least your suffering, was at last out of my sight. I plunged myself into academic success and a profession divorced from the needs of my heart. Our already fragmented family finally disintegrated at your death, each of us confined to our separate private prisons, reeling with our separate private pains, and unable to break down our walls to finally begin to find each other. The social stigma around mention of suicide cemented us apart from then on. My parents gave us to understand that we were not to talk of you.

In the end, years later, beginning to experience alarming feelings of being so anxious I could not sleep, I went for psychological counselling. Your hospital file was accessed and I was told some of the details of your death. It was your Doctor's words of comfort to my parents that enraged me beyond belief and finally told me that my heart had been broken:

'Rose was a very sweet child but was heavily handicapped in the struggle for existence by inner psychological difficulties. Life would have been very difficult for her and much as I regret what has happened, I think you should take comfort in the fact that she is at peace at last in the arms of her Saviour.'

When you were finally given a grave-stone many years after your death, it said simply your name and 'safe in the arms of Jesus'. I felt like attacking the gravestone. I was beside myself.

Was I to conclude from the doctor's consolations that you were better off dead, that the arms of Jesus was the only place of safety for you, you who had lain safely in my arms so many nights of our childhood? The official line was to be that your troubles were all inner and no awkward questions asked. But your death and the reasons for it could not be so neatly erased from my mind. The best part of my life has been spent in unravelling the path that took you there.

The heavy black mantle of guilt for your pain which had descended on my shoulders so early on in my life now enveloped me completely. You had in childhood jealousy told me I always spoiled things for you. Part of me accepted this as the truth. So when you eventually took your life, my sense of responsibility was so overwhelming, I did not let it into my consciousness. Instead it drove my life for many years, leading me into punishing relationships and unable to stay with loving partners. Also, of course my life was scarred by sudden endings and deaths.

Unable at first to feel my own sense of guilt, I ascribed it firstly to our abusive parents, then to you yourself, for lacking moral backbone. It was easy to blame our parents, they had been abusive, and it was also easy to blame you. Society had a dim view of suicides and you should have toughened up like me. It was impossible for me to admit how much I felt I was to blame.

Yet all along I had sensed underneath that our parents couldn't be held responsible for your death. I knew enough of their own childhood torments to realize how scarred they were, and how unwittingly they acted out on us. Moreover, our father was irrevocably damaged by untreated traumatic stress disorder due to the horror that was World War ll. He spent several months in a mental hospital at the end of the war but never properly recovered. Current estimates suggest that a staggering proportion of men involved in combat suffer severe psychological damage unless given urgent expert treatment. These men are mostly fathers at some point in their lives. My father's own dad came home in 1918 to die slowly from gas in his lungs in front of his 4-year old son. So nobody taught my father how to be a Dad. And in a society rightly termed the State of Atrocity by feminist philosopher, Mary Daly, violence is part of the daily currency. Thus it is no surprise for me now that our 'cultural' conditioning leads many of us to use violence on the bodies of others, or on our own.

I could no longer blame our parents. I can no longer blame you. You, my older sister, always seemed as if you should have known the answers. But you were only twenty when you took your own life. When I witnessed my own daughter at twenty, I saw how young and vulnerable you were. I can feel compassion for you now. How could I have blamed you?

I blamed you because I did not want to admit how much I blamed myself. Yet the evidence of the way I lived my life since your death screams it out. I couldn't stop your death, I must have let you down, or worse still, been somebody so horrid that you wanted to get away from me altogether; I who was only thirteen when you started suicide attempts and sixteen when you died; I who tried to do my utmost to cheer you up, to listen to your weepy outpourings of self-hatred. And there was nobody around for me on whom to offload my anguish even if I had been able to admit it. So for years my guilt crippled my life.

It is only as I have acknowledged and felt my own pain and experienced for myself the hell of depression and of how you might have felt that I can see, Rosie, that nobody in our immediate world was directly responsible for your death. I can bewail the tragedy that there were only damaging medical resources available at that time for you.

But for me the ultimate truth is that, in this barbaric social order, built on a hierarchy of violence, you were one of the obvious casualties. The human condition, as it is euphemistically called, should not in itself breed such despair and self-destructiveness. There are faceless ones responsible for human misery, those who in the nineteenth century profited from the slave employment of children forced to work in dangerous mills from 4.00 a.m. and dying at age thirteen exhausted. Today millions of children's lives in Asia and elsewhere are broken as they are systematically exploited as child prostitutes - somebody is making money out of this. In the 'civilized' world billions of pounds of illegal trade make the sale of child pornography a top contributor to criminal coffers, along with drugs and armaments sales. The bodies of young men and others are mutilated in senseless conflicts which could have been resolved rationally.

In order that a handful of people on this planet can live off the fat of the land, the rest of us are condemned to accept a way of life that is responsible now for the vast army of slow suicides of drug addicted youth, for the perpetual deaths of millions starving, and for the suffocation of the life-breath of our earthly home, near her last polluted gasp. These few have been raised and educated to be morally and emotionally crippled – they are enjoying the spoils of such a back-ground but cannot be held to be individually responsible - they are themselves products of an elitist rogue regime. Raise children as they are raised and we get what we get.

Life has been brutish, short and nasty for the vast proportion of humanity for a long time. I hold that this is not an inevitable condition, but one that is susceptible to social change. The question remains as to whether those in power can be required to change in time, before we descend helter-skelter into a profit--fuelled ecological catastrophe. Your death, Rosie, and the questions around its causes, have radicalized me. My anger at your death is not now directed at you, my poor sister, but at those who still profit knowingly from exploitation.

So I will not be ashamed of you and be silent about your end. I speak of you now to help break down these walls of shaming isolation, for myself and others. I want my human family to remake itself. I want to belong like I have never belonged, but to a society that is worthy of my loyalty.

So where does that leave me with you, sweet sister, the sister I cast into the nether reaches of my soul for so long? How do I end this account, draw a line around your life and death, and say 'This is past, over and done with?' How many times over the years have I straddled that door with you in an effort to stop you doing the unthinkable, tried to rewrite your end so that I can again follow in your footsteps through life? At the time of your death, in spite of being lied to, I knew that you had killed yourself out of sheer misery and despair. I promised you that I would try to be happy, to be happy for the part of you that lived on in me. But that promise propelled me instead down, down to touch rock-bottom of the pain of your chosen death. Gentle access to that awful space was barred for me for many years by the poisonous shaming surrounding suicide. It has taken me years to begin to feel moments of happiness again.

And when at long last I experience sweet moments in life, they immediately conjure you up, my first and most abiding love, standing laughing with the frost aglow in your hair. Those moments of happiness, hard-wrested from the knot of pain woven tight around our family nexus, bring you back to me, standing beside me, as you were when we were little. I did not follow you into the oblivion of death, or whatever death holds. For your chosen death has impelled me to uncover the pain I share with you, to make myself a whole human being, to support other victims of abuse and to use my woundedness to fight for its eradication. - and to create safe spaces for all of Earth's children.

I have felt my own despair and depression over the years, Rosie. And the fact that I chose to go on living is not to say you were wrong to choose to die. There is nothing now for me to forgive. Belatedly, I am trying to say what I couldn't say at the time to you, that I understand.

On your last complete day on earth, you confessed to our father that you were afraid of him. That took so much courage. And in honour of you, I will ceaselessly drag your broken body from the unspeakable crossroads to which society has consigned it. You are not beyond the pale. You belong to a community and your death should have been honoured, simply as it was. You died because you wanted to at the time, that took sheer courage. Life as it was for you was unbearable and the conditions of existence at present on this planet make it unbearable for billions of others. You are not alone. The official verdict on your death certificate was instantaneous death by hanging. My verdict is slow death by social strangulation of your precious vibrant energy.

May you rest in peace but the struggle for liberation of human beings, for the life that you should have lived, live on.